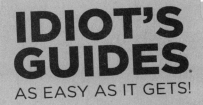

IDIOT'S GUIDES.
AS EASY AS IT GETS!

The Chia Seed Diet

by Bud E. Smith, Paul Plotkin, and Joseph Ewing, RD, LDN

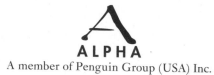

ALPHA

A member of Penguin Group (USA) Inc.

ALPHA BOOKS

Published by Penguin Group (USA) Inc.

Penguin Group (USA) Inc., 375 Hudson Street, New York, New York 10014, USA • Penguin Group (Canada), 90 Eglinton Avenue East, Suite 700, Toronto, Ontario M4P 2Y3, Canada (a division of Pearson Penguin Canada Inc.) • Penguin Books Ltd., 80 Strand, London WC2R 0RL, England • Penguin Ireland, 25 St. Stephen's Green, Dublin 2, Ireland (a division of Penguin Books Ltd.) • Penguin Group (Australia), 250 Camberwell Road, Camberwell, Victoria 3124, Australia (a division of Pearson Australia Group Pty. Ltd.) • Penguin Books India Pvt. Ltd., 11 Community Centre, Panchsheel Park, New Delhi—110 017, India • Penguin Group (NZ), 67 Apollo Drive, Rosedale, North Shore, Auckland 1311, New Zealand (a division of Pearson New Zealand Ltd.) • Penguin Books (South Africa) (Pty.) Ltd., 24 Sturdee Avenue, Rosebank, Johannesburg 2196, South Africa • Penguin Books Ltd., Registered Offices: 80 Strand, London WC2R 0RL, England

International Standard Book Number: 978-1-61564-441-4
Library of Congress Catalog Card Number: 2013948133

16   15   14   8   7   6   5   4   3   2   1

Interpretation of the printing code: The rightmost number of the first series of numbers is the year of the book's printing; the rightmost number of the second series of numbers is the number of the book's printing. For example, a printing code of 14-1 shows that the first printing occurred in 2014.

Printed in the United States of America

Note: This publication contains the opinions and ideas of its authors. It is intended to provide helpful and informative material on the subject matter covered. It is sold with the understanding that the authors and publisher are not engaged in rendering professional services in the book. If the reader requires personal assistance or advice, a competent professional should be consulted. The authors and publisher specifically disclaim any responsibility for any liability, loss, or risk, personal or otherwise, which is incurred as a consequence, directly or indirectly, of the use and application of any of the contents of this book.

Most Alpha books are available at special quantity discounts for bulk purchases for sales promotions, premiums, fundraising, or educational use. Special books, or book excerpts, can also be created to fit specific needs. For details, write: Special Markets, Alpha Books, 375 Hudson Street, New York, NY 10014.

Publisher: *Mike Sanders*
Executive Managing Editor: *Billy Fields*
Executive Acquisitions Editor: *Lori Cates Hand*
Development Editor: *Kayla Dugger*
Production Editor: *Jana M. Stefanciosa*

Cover Designer: *Laura Merriman*
Book Designer: *William Thomas*
Indexer: *Tonya Heard*
Layout: *Ayanna Lacey*
Proofreader: *Gene Redding*

Contents

Introduction

Chia and chia seeds mean many things to many different people. A few might not even be aware that they've ever heard of chia. Many others may think of Chia Pets, whether through the famous "Ch-ch-ch-ch-chia!" TV ads that launched them into public awareness or the novelty versions like Chia Smurfs, Chia President Obama, or Chia Governor Romney. But the way some people know about chia—and the one more in line with the purpose of this book—is as a superfood.

Chia is the single best and most effective food around to help you with your weight-loss and weight-management goals. There's nothing like chia for helping you feel more full with less food and for avoiding the swings between hunger and feeling stuffed that are so much a part of life on a Western diet with lots of processed foods and fast food. Chia is also at or near the top for a whole host of other purposes, such as better nutrition, improved digestion, a healthier heart, and better endurance. This is the promise chia holds, and this book is built on that promise.

There's nothing overhyped or "woo-woo" about this book. Chia won't automatically give you the strength of an Aztec warrior or the endurance of a Pueblo Indian message runner. Nor will it spiritually enlighten you. But chia will help you feel better and eat better—and perhaps give you a little boost toward gaining all those other good things as well.

How This Book Is Organized

This book is divided into four parts, each dealing with a different aspect of adding chia to your daily diet.

Part 1, Introducing Chia, explains why chia seeds evolved to be such a powerful superfood for people and the many benefits they can give you. This part also spells out how chia works in your body to aid weight loss, weight management, and digestion; give you high levels of energy; and more.

Part 2, Bringing Chia into Your Life, discusses how chia complements other diets, whether vegan or vegetarian, low-carb, gluten-free, paleo, or something else. You also learn how to get chia into your diet, whether mixed in via seeds and gel or as an egg or flour substitute. We also give you information on other chia products you can buy; you get a rundown of everything from foods with chia already in them to personal-care products that include it. We close this part with a shopping list to help you start the diet off right.

Part 3, Using the Chia Seed Diet, shows you how to integrate chia into the different parts of your life that are affected by how you eat, such as your eating habits with family and friends, your diet while traveling, and much more. This part also has solid suggestions for integrating exercise into your chia diet lifestyle, allowing you to take advantage of chia's ability to help you maintain a high energy level long after you've finished a meal. We also provide two-week meal plans you can use as a blueprint for planning your meals.

Part 4, Chia Recipes, is in some ways the heart of the book. It contains scores of handy, delicious, easy-to-use recipes covering every part of your day and every part of your diet. You can use these recipes to help you plan your meals, whether it's a dinner with side dishes or a quick, healthy snack. It also helps combine theory and action: With these recipes, you learn how chia feels in all parts of your diet and get ideas for how to integrate chia into a vast array of other things you eat and drink.

At the end of the book, you find a glossary and a list of resources. The resources include books and websites about the benefits of chia and even how you can grow your own chia plants.

Extras

Throughout the chapters of the book, four types of additional information, set apart in sidebars, can help you better understand the information and enrich your learning process:

DEFINITION

These sidebars include specialized dietary and chia-related terms you may encounter when you begin this diet.

SEEDS OF CHANGE

These sidebars provide tips and other ideas that can help you implement the chia seed diet in the easiest way possible.

CHIA CAUTION

These sidebars point out potential pitfalls to avoid as you learn more about chia.

FOOD FOR THOUGHT

In these sidebars, you'll find quotes from diet experts and researchers that enrich your reading experience, give you different perspectives, and point you toward other books you might want to read.

Acknowledgments

Our appreciation goes first to the many people who worked hard to understand, preserve, extend, and repopularize aspects of Native American culture, not least of which is the tiny yet powerful chia seed.

We also want to thank the many people who taught us to eat, cook, and share better. In some cases, this learning has meant challenging a lot of conventional wisdom. We're happy to share the results with you.

Trademarks

All terms mentioned in this book that are known to be or are suspected of being trademarks or service marks have been appropriately capitalized. Alpha Books and Penguin Group (USA) Inc. cannot attest to the accuracy of this information. Use of a term in this book should not be regarded as affecting the validity of any trademark or service mark.

Medical Disclaimer

The publisher is not responsible for your specific health or medical needs that may require medical supervision. Neither the publisher nor the authors are engaged in rendering professional advice or services to the individual reader. The ideas, procedures, and suggestions contained in this book are not intended as a substitute for consulting with your physician. Neither the authors nor the publisher is responsible for any adverse reactions to the remedies contained in this book and neither shall be liable for any loss or damage allegedly arising from any information or suggestion in this book.

Introducing Chia

People aren't robots who blindly follow instructions, especially not when it comes to their diet. Changing dietary habits is one of the biggest challenges you can face. So this part of the book, about why chia seeds are so powerful in helping you meet your health and weight-loss goals, may be the most important part of the book.

This part tells you how chia got its start as a major food source for Native American cultures— and how it was suppressed for centuries after Europeans arrived. You also get information on what the chia plant is like and how the chia seed came to be as powerful a superfood as any, if not more so.

In this part, you also learn about the benefits of chia for weight loss and weight management, improved nutrition, better digestion, and endurance.

The Origins and Benefits of Chia

Chia seeds are tiny seeds, so small they look like specks rather than fully developed seeds. The chia plant is a kind of sage that grows in hot desert environments, native to central Mexico and the American Southwest. To thrive in this harsh environment, chia seeds are packed with nutrients and good fats. You can sprinkle them on soups and salads, mix them in with gravies and dressings, stir them into smoothies, and more. Chia seeds have many beneficial effects on health while reducing your appetite; in many ways, chia seeds are the most "super" of superfoods.

Like many traditional foods, chia has been largely forgotten for hundreds of years, but now, it's making a huge comeback.

This chapter describes chia's origins in some detail to help you understand how important chia can be in your diet—and why we need it so badly today. We also tell you why we need to pay extra attention to our diets to achieve the strength and health we all want. We then explain how we got chia back from the obscurity in which it languished for 500 years.

In This Chapter

- Chia's origins and uses
- How the human diet has changed over time
- Why we need chia and other superfoods
- Today's chia renaissance

An Ancient Food with Modern Benefits

Chia is amazing. It comes to us from the Mayans, Aztecs, Incas, and other ancient Native American cultures. These people and their descendants have raised chia for more than 5,000 years.

FOOD FOR THOUGHT

Chia was one of the primary food crops of Native Americans and was highly valued— so much so that chia seeds were used as money.

The word *chia* means "strength" in the Mayan language, and making you stronger is one of the primary benefits of chia. Among Native Americans, chia was particularly known for its ability to help people run all day without tiring.

But chia is not just for endurance running or strength training. Chia helps to solve many of the problems of modern diets and modern lifestyles. It contains omega-3 fatty acids that are all too rare in the modern diet, where the less healthy omega-6 acids predominate. Chia seeds are full of nutrients, such as calcium, zinc, and more. A real partner in the struggle against being over-weight, diabetes, and heart disease, chia is a true superfood: a strength booster, nutritional supplement, diet aid, and medicine, all in one tiny seed.

We in the developed world tend to celebrate the virtues of Western lifestyles and knowledge over "primitive" cultures. However, there is considerable evidence that many Native Americans ate better before European colonization than after.

The diet of the Aztecs included fish and turkey; beans and corn, which together make a complete protein; and fruit and vegetables. They also ate grains and grainlike seeds, including amaranth, bulgur, quinoa, and lots of chia. The Aztecs even used chia seeds for oil.

Compare this to the typical diet of the modern American. The American diet tends to rely heavily on processed foods, many of which include refined grains and sugars. For protein, Americans more often eat meat than beans and corn. Unlike the Aztecs, modern Americans consume beef and pork, which are higher in fat than other meats. Whole fruits and vegetables don't feature as prominently in the typical American diet as they need to. Instead, Americans tend to eat a lot of breads, pasta, and other wheat-based foods.

Although these are generalizations and certainly not true of all Americans, it's safe to say that the foods most Americans regularly consume are higher in fat, sugar, and sodium than the foods eaten by the ancient Aztecs. The consequences of the American diet can be seen in the rise of many health issues, including heart disease, diabetes, and obesity.

The good news is that a richer diet with more variety and more superfoods is very much in the reach of most Americans. This superior diet is arguably cheaper on a food cost basis and inarguably healthier—with lower associated medical costs—than the mainstream American diet.

How Native Americans Used Chia

Native Americans in Mexico began using chia more than 5,000 years ago. The Teotihuacan, Toltec, and Aztec civilizations used it, and it was used heavily by the Aztecs in particular.

The Aztecs used chia in many ways. They ate it directly, added it to other foods, and used it to make drinks (see Part 4). They also ground chia seeds to make flour and pressed it for oil. In many forms, such as flour, chia was and is easily preserved—a crucial positive in all human cultures before refrigeration.

 FOOD FOR THOUGHT

Chia was also used as a base material for medicines and nutritional foods and drinks—what we would consider a supplement today.

One key usage of chia by the Aztecs, which led to its suppression, was its involvement in religious ceremonies. Beyond being widely used and respected, chia was offered to the gods. The invading Spanish took note of this and deliberately suppressed the use of chia, stamping out its cultivation wherever they could.

Although chia use reached its peak with the Aztecs, it was widely used throughout the Americas. The Inca famously used runners to send messages over long distances, and these athletes used chia as a compact food source and to make a kind of energy drink. In other parts of North America, native people used chia as a food source during long trading trips, and they made a poultice from chia to apply to wounds—even severe wounds, such as gunshot wounds. We still don't have a complete understanding of all the ways in which chia was used in Native American cultures.

The Disappearance of Native Foods and Culture

America is famous for being a melting pot of cultures and influences from all over the world. Europe is known for being cosmopolitan. Yet there is very little influence from Native American cultures in either society. Why is this? In particular, why is something as obviously positive as chia only recently getting attention, more than 500 years after Europeans came to the Americas?

For starters, the influence of the Aztecs, and of all Native Americans, was diminished by the impact of disease brought by early European settlers. The lack of sanitary conditions in European cities and towns led to plagues and disease that, in the 1300s alone killed an estimated one third of the people in Europe.

The plague was followed by other diseases to which the Europeans developed resistance but not immunity—so they brought these diseases with them wherever they went. So when Europeans landed in the formerly isolated Americas, the disease impact was huge. More than half the population of the Americas died within a few decades, most without ever seeing a white man.

Because the Aztecs and other native people died so quickly and in such great numbers, there were too few to carry on their traditions and lifestyle strongly.

Despite the huge population losses suffered by the native people at the time of European settlement, there are still many Central and South American countries that are predominantly Native American. However, in these countries, Native American languages, cultures, and traditions have historically been suppressed.

Like many aspects of Native American culture, chia was nearly lost. Spanish settlers mostly halted its cultivation, and it survived only in some isolated areas of Mexico.

The Evolution of the Human Diet

It's easier to understand the many benefits of chia if you see some of the ways in which our modern lifestyles contribute to specific health problems that our ancestors didn't have. In fact, the health and lifestyle problems many of us want to avoid today are almost the opposite of the health problems people have faced for most of human history.

Learning about how human lives have changed over time will motivate you to make changes in your own diet and lifestyle that will help you to be strong, healthy, vital, and lively well into the future. One of the easiest and most beneficial changes you can make is to adjust your diet to include much more chia.

The Diet of Early Man

People evolved in what is now Africa as hunter-gatherers who lived in small tribes. As people evolved, the climate and the environments in which they lived changed many times. It was their flexibility and adaptability that allowed them to compete with other creatures that had thicker fur, tougher hides, sharper teeth, and longer claws—that were stronger, moved faster, or had other advantages over humans.

The key development that made humanity and, later, today's technologies possible was the mastery of fire. No other creature has ever tamed fire. For early people, fire meant warmth, safety, and the ability to cook food. Although there's a lot of controversy around old fossils and old fire pits, it looks as if pre-humans first used fire more than a million years ago.

Our early ancestors ate a lot of fruit, nuts, and foliage and not much meat. With fire and the later development of weapons and hunting techniques, they added more meat to the fruit, nuts, and foliage. This created a relatively rich diet that seems to have allowed humans to become fully upright and to develop bigger brains. Early humans moved fully out of the trees, invented language, developed complex social networks, and steadily improved their tools and weapons.

Eventually, humans began to spread beyond what is now Africa, perhaps in several different waves. It is believed that people settled first in the Middle East, then South Asia and Southeast Asia. The ancestors of aborigines reached Australia about 50,000 years ago, and the ancestors of today's Native Americans reached the Americas only about 15,000 years ago. They arrived by crossing a land and ice bridge from Siberia to Alaska at the end of the last Ice Age.

 FOOD FOR THOUGHT

There is some evidence that people from Southeast Asia reached and settled the Americas first but were overwhelmed by Northeast Asians—the ancestors of today's Native Americans—who arrived at the end of the last Ice Age.

It was Native Americans who found and nurtured chia and then made it a centerpiece of their daily lives and culture.

The Agriculture Explosion

The early hunter-gatherers moved a lot; both hunting and gathering involve lots of walking and running. A fully grown man who spends his day sitting may only burn about 2,000 calories, but if he were to spend his day walking, he could burn 500 calories an hour. An active hunter or gatherer might need to eat two or three times as much as most people today just to keep going.

In eating so much food—all of it "natural," little of it processed or preserved—early humans worked their digestive systems hard. They also had the opportunity to get lots of nutrients, including phytochemicals and micronutrients. While people suffered from many health problems that are easily curable today, many people were tall and strong, and some modern problems, such as tooth decay, were very rare.

However, around the time that people reached the Americas, the best—and worst—thing in the history of humanity happened: the invention of large-scale agriculture.

People had always used cereal grains, rice, and other wild grains as a part of their diets. But fruits, nuts, grasses, and meats made up the majority of what people ate most of the time. The retreat of the glaciers led to thousands of years of stable climate, and the stable climate led people to undertake large-scale experiments with growing staple crops in a settled area—usually a river delta—over long periods of time.

How We Eat Today

Agriculture led to exploding populations and to modern civilization. It also led to poor diets, with people subsisting on large quantities of a single staple. Hunting was often reserved for the nobility, and farm animals were few and precious. For most people, protein and many other nutrients were scarce. The average height of people decreased, largely due to the lack of protein. Tooth decay exploded due to poor diets.

In the developed world today, people again have access to a wide variety of food if they want it. But modern agriculture tends toward monocultures—a few varieties of each crop, rather than the rich variety found in nature. Mechanized farming also depletes the soil; while results vary, one study in the United States found that several varieties of apples had about one quarter fewer nutrients today than they had 50 years ago.

Meat is plentiful in most people's diets, perhaps too much so. Most people get enough protein, but it comes with fats and harmful chemicals fed to livestock. The animals have bland diets full of chemicals and drugs, so meat and milk are lacking in nutrition and have the residues of the chemicals and drugs in them.

To compound the problem, people in the developed world are largely sedentary. People drive instead of walking, which makes for a huge reduction in calories burned. People do eat less than before, but not enough less, so excess weight, obesity, and diabetes are big health concerns.

Dangerous Consequences

One consequence of our modern diet and lifestyle is an increase in the number of people diagnosed with type 1 *diabetes*. This disease is becoming epidemic in America, and many other developed countries are also seeing a rapid increase. Unlike type 1 diabetes, people are not born with type 2 diabetes. The disease used to be called "adult-onset" diabetes, because it took years of an unhealthy diet before a person would develop it. Now, many of us have the wrong type of diet from such an early age that teenagers and even children are seen with type 2 diabetes.

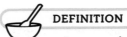

DEFINITION

A person who suffers from **diabetes** has problems processing and storing sugar. Sufferers may need injections of insulin to help their bodies process sugar. There are two types of diabetes: type 1 diabetes, which begins at birth; and type 2 diabetes, which begins later and has been linked to obesity.

Type 2 diabetes is associated with diets that are high in sugar and lacking in fiber and nutrients. These diets can cause people to become overweight or obese, conditions that are in turn strongly linked to type 2 diabetes. The fate of a diabetic person can be awful; weight seems impossible to control for many diabetics, and health problems follow.

Type 2 diabetes is often treated with drugs to control blood sugar, but making aggressive life-style changes can also make a world of difference. Many formerly diabetic people have returned to normal blood sugar levels and weight and have little or no need for drugs—all due to making significant changes in diet and exercise patterns (see Chapter 4 for more on chia as a diabetes fighter).

How Superfoods Can Help

Humanity has used its intelligence—and a great deal of hard work—to create a world where food is relatively cheap and plentiful in many countries. The average amount of income that the average American or European spends on food, for instance, has dropped steadily for decades. People in America a hundred years ago used to spend about 50 percent of their money on food; now they spend about 10 percent.

We live in a time when food is plentiful for many people. While humanity was evolving, it was often a struggle to get enough food to fuel a strenuous lifestyle. Now, the opposite problem appears: There's too much food, much of it not very good for us, and little physical effort in our daily routines to work it off. In fact, our bodies are so bored with the lack of movement, and easy indoor environments, that food can become an interesting distraction.

Also, because our food is bland, we don't get the signal to our brains that we've had enough. Instead, we just keep eating until our stomachs are so stuffed that the message finally gets through: enough!

These are side effects of the world we've developed that we have to watch out for. To live a long and healthy life, you need to use your intelligence and good sense to avoid these pitfalls. Even a small amount of attention and care to your diet, plus a moderate amount of exercise, can be a huge help.

If you want to be particularly healthy—to have an active or athletic lifestyle, feeling good much or all of the time, and to have your food and drink be a source of joy—then thinking about what you eat and drink needs to be part of your daily approach to life.

This is where superfoods in general, and chia in particular, come in. Superfoods are highly dense in energy and full of nutrition. Superfoods are usually whole foods without chemicals and other harmful additives.

Many foods are described as superfoods—and many have become quite popular. Salmon, for instance, has a high percentage of omega-3 fatty acids, which are considered to be good for your heart. Yogurt—especially low-fat Greek yogurt, without added sugar—has beneficial enzymes and makes you feel full with few calories. Sweet potatoes have more nutrition than white potatoes and are quite filling; their rich flavor reduces the temptation to load them up with butter and sour cream.

Superfoods allow you to get the concentrated nutrition you need without taking in many calories. If you're active, superfoods give you the extra boost you need to support increased exertion and recovery from exercise.

Superfoods can have an almost medicinal effect. Many of the health problems that are common today—diabetes, heart disease, and cancer—are linked to bland diets heavy in processed foods. Shifting your diet toward superfoods and away from mainstream diets gives you the opportunity to avoid these problems.

Why We Need Chia

Chia is almost a super-superfood. We are lucky it was discovered and used so widely and so well by Native Americans, then rescued and popularized in the West.

We'll go into much more detail in this book about chia's many benefits, but here are a few highlights—in the context of the problems with our modern food system.

The first is that chia forms a kind of gel in your stomach. Chia seeds are oily—which is a quality you have to work with when you add it to foods. When you eat chia, that oiliness creates a matrix that settles in your gut, making you feel full. With chia, you digest your food more slowly.

Chia thus helps to solve one of the biggest problems people have with modern diets: the tendency to overeat. Including chia in your diet throughout the day reduces your desire for food and buffers the impact of the food you do have.

This quality of chia has many benefits, moving chia to the top of the heap of superfoods. Eating less food—because you feel full sooner—and digesting it more slowly, because of the chia-based matrix that forms, are wonderful contributions for those recovering from diabetes. Chia can be so effective for weight loss that it's been called "*lap band surgery* in a seed."

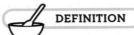 **DEFINITION**

Lap band surgery is an operation in which a physical band is put around the stomach. This forces the patient to limit how much he or she eats. This surgery is much more common in America than elsewhere. Governor Chris Christie of New Jersey is among the many people, famous and not so famous, who have had lap band surgery.

With chia, you can take in less sugary, fatty food and still feel full—that's why chia is compared to lap band surgery. And, unlike with lap band surgery, the food you do eat digests more slowly, reducing the peaks in blood sugar that characterize diabetes.

Chia seeds are packed with nutrients that help your body function optimally. These nutrients include the following:

- Protein, which reduces the need to eat meat

- Iron, which is also otherwise hard to get without meat

- Omega-3 fatty acids, the "good" kind of fat, which balance the omega-6 fatty acids found in many other foods

- Fiber, which is good for digestion and actually cleans out your gut. Fiber also helps your body to absorb all the nutrients in your food more efficiently

- Calcium, which is especially important for women who otherwise might have trouble maintaining strong, dense bones

- Antioxidants, which reduce damage at a cellular level—damage associated with cancer and other health problems

Taken together, these attributes can help lower your cholesterol, which is a major predictor of heart disease.

All of this is important, but it's also only one side of chia. Not only does chia help avoid health problems; it's known as a strong contributor to athletic performance, which is one of the main ways the Maya and Aztecs used it. Better athletic performance can spice up your life when you're out jogging, playing sports, even in the bedroom. And the more physical activity of all kinds you engage in, the healthier you're likely to be.

So chia can be part of a virtuous circle for your life and health, making it easier to feel good, look good, and enjoy yourself.

Chia Seeds and Endurance

Chia seeds were well known among Native Americans for their ability to boost endurance. Aztec warriors, said to be among the fiercest the world has ever known, used them to keep going in battle.

The Tarahumara Indians of Mexico are famous for running hundreds of miles with little rest or food, and chia is a mainstay for them. The Tarahumara, and their use of chia, are featured in Christopher McDougall's book *Born to Run: A Hidden Tribe, Superathletes, and the Greatest Race the World Has Never Seen.*

Chia is now becoming a mainstay for runners and other endurance athletes in our current culture. They are touted as "God's gift to endurance runners" and "the Muhammad Ali of nutrition." Baltimore Ravens running back Ray Rice, who is well known for his healthy diet and lifestyle, sees chia seeds as giving him a boost.

You will also find chia seeds among the foods recommended to increase sexual performance and enjoyment. People who have no interest in other athletic endeavors still want to feel like champions in their intimate lives, and chia is famous for its contribution here, too.

The Chia Renaissance

The comeback of chia, which continues today, is an amazing story.

After it was nearly exterminated by the Spanish, chia use in Mexico and a few other countries continued on a very small scale. It was used to make chia fresca (see Chapter 12 for a recipe), a drink with medicinal and religious significance. However, very little chia was grown or sold on any kind of commercial basis.

The next move for chia was its use for something truly trivial: the Chia Pet. Chia Pets are clay figures that come in a variety of animal shapes. Where an animal might have a coat of fur, the figures are scored with grooves that can hold chia seeds. Watering a Chia Pet quickly gives it a rich coat of green "wool" as the chia seeds sprout. Chia Pets are still sold; however, the initial burst of popularity for Chia Pets was not enough to bring it into widespread usage as a food. Still, Chia Pets are a testament to the vitality of chia seeds, which can handle the harsh treatment of being kept in a dark box for months, or even years, and then sprouting reliably when needed.

 FOOD FOR THOUGHT

At chiapet.com, you can purchase Chia Pets, refill chia seeds for Chia Pets, buy a chia seed growing kit, get branded chia seeds, get softgel tablets with chia in them, and more.

Then, in the early 1990s, a campaign began in Argentina to revive traditional and local plants. Ricardo Ayerza is an Argentinian biochemist who helped lead this revival; he worked with American Wayne Coates. They first introduced chia into chicken feed, and better-tasting eggs were the result. This introduced the use of chia for various animal husbandry and veterinary purposes that continues today; many pet owners feed chia to their pets.

Chia use has exploded, but from a very small base. The many benefits of chia—described throughout this book—have gotten attention all over the map and from many different interest groups: diabetics, dieters, vegetarians, athletes, and many others.

Chia use continues to grow but has yet to become mainstream. Given the great need for all that chia has to offer—perhaps most spectacularly in diets for fighting diabetes—it can be hoped that the chia revival is a long way from its peak and that it won't be over as long as people eat, run, and otherwise enjoy and use food.

The Least You Need to Know

- Chia was originally grown and used by the Aztecs, Mayans, and other Native Americans.
- *Chia* means "strength" in the Mayan language and is recognized for aiding endurance.
- Our modern diets and lifestyles can cause a variety of health problems, some of which can be remedied by in part by consuming more chia.
- Chia slows digestion, which is helpful for those with type 2 diabetes.
- Chia is on most lists of "superfoods" and contains many beneficial nutrients.

Chia in Depth

Most of the information you encounter about chia focuses on its health benefits, plus a few highlights of the chia plant and the seed itself. We think it's important for you to know more about it—how it grows, the structure of the seed, and what it tastes like.

Chia is fascinating. It's also complex; people have been cultivating chia for thousands of years, so it's been adapted somewhat to human use. We may never know exactly what the original chia plant was like before people started tending it, selecting the qualities that made it most useful to them.

We want chia to be part of your diet for the rest of your life, and for you to be empowered to find new and creative ways to use it. In order to do that, you'll need to know as much about chia as possible, starting with the plant.

In This Chapter

- In-depth information about the chia plant
- Considering calories when adding chia to your diet
- What does chia taste like?

The Chia Plant

The chia seeds you buy at the grocery store are the product of the chia plant, *Salvia hispanica.* Imagine a bushy herb up to 3 feet tall, with leaves 2 to 3 inches long and 1 to 2 inches wide. Chia plants have white or purple flowers that come out of a spike at the end of a stem.

Chia seeds are the part of the plant we eat for nutritional benefit. They are tiny ovals about 1 millimeter long, which is less than $^1/_{16}$ inch. They can be black, white, or multihued. There really isn't much difference between the various colors of the seeds.

Why Are Seeds so Great?

Seeds are fantastic! Seeds of various sorts come up over and over again in looking out for super-foods and other healthy foods. Chia and flax are two top superfoods that are seeds. Nuts are a type of seed, just one with a particularly hard shell.

Seeds are some of the best superfoods because they pack everything the young plant needs into the smallest package. This includes three key elements, as you can see in the following figure:

- **Dormant embryo:** This is the part of the seed that grows into a fully capable plant.

- **Endosperm:** The endosperm stores nutrients for the embryo. It gives the embryo a boost.

- **Seed coat:** This is the shell around the seed to keep out the elements—including the digestive juices of any animal that might ingest the seed.

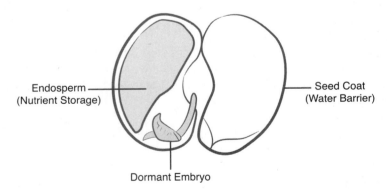

Endosperm
(Nutrient Storage)

Seed Coat
(Water Barrier)

Dormant Embryo

Seeds are simple: a baby plant and its food.

All seeds are packed with nutrition. They contain the nutrients that are most needed by the developing plant and least likely to be available in the soil right around the plant.

Chia's Strategies for Survival

All seeds are packed with nutrients, but there are two factors that make chia even more powerful than most: wind and animal dispersal, and a harsh environment.

 FOOD FOR THOUGHT

The chia plant's strategies for survival made its seed what it is today—a true superfood for human health. Native Americans recognized this and made chia a big part of their diet; today's mainstream American culture is only starting to catch on.

Wind and Animal Dispersal

Over time, plants have developed different "strategies" for spreading their seeds. Seeds designed to be dispersed by wind have physical features to help them travel. For instance, dandelion seeds have "wings" that help them get caught by the wind and carried a long way. Other seeds grow inside fruits and vegetables. Animals, including humans, eat the fruits and vegetables, along with the seeds they contain. Some of the seeds are digested by the animal, but others pass through undigested. The animal gets the benefit of nutrients, fiber, and calories it needs, and the seed is spread in the animal's droppings.

The chia seed has evolved to be so small that it can be spread by both wind and animal dispersal. It's so tiny that it can get picked up by the wind, eaten by an animal that happens to eat the flower, or picked up on the paw or wing of a passing animal or bird.

Chia plants also give nectar to bees, butterflies, and birds. The seeds are so small that they easily attach to the sticky nectar and to the creature that eats the nectar. The seeds are also eaten directly as food by birds, mammals, and insects.

There's a bit of a trade-off here: The only species that have much incentive to eat the seeds are species that can digest them, to get the nutritional benefit. So while some of the seeds are digested, enough have to survive and be passed out of the animal intact to make the whole effort worthwhile for the plant. The chia seed is just tough enough so that many, but not all, of the seeds survive the trip through the digestive tract.

The Harsh Desert Environment

The desert environment plays a big part in making chia a superfood. Millions of years of evolution have packed a lot of "learning" into the plant's genetic code. Each chia plant creates seeds that have a good chance of surviving in the environment that chia is adapted to—the desert.

Its small size makes it easily carried by wind and likely to be eaten by small desert creatures. However, this means a lot of nutrients must be packed into a very small package. In many cases, it won't have the benefit of being surrounded by natural fertilizer from an animal's dung. And it's in a very harsh environment, the hot deserts of Central America. Among Earth's varied environments, only polar environments are harsher than deserts. The word *desert,* after all, comes from the same root as the word *deserted,* or empty.

Chia seeds, like many seeds, are oily, as oils retain water against evaporation and contain fats that are full of nutrition for the young plant. The desert soil is very unlikely to have much to sustain the new, tiny chia plant—and the chia seed is unusually small—so the oils in a chia seed are especially dense and nutritious.

Oils, as many of us have learned the hard way, tend to go rancid. To guard against this tendency, chia seeds are rich in antioxidants, which help prevent oils from going rancid. They also happen to help people have healthy hearts and immune systems and fight cancer.

Chia seeds are rich in omega-3 fatty acids, which are energy intensive for the parent plant to create and very valuable for the young plant. They also have a very high amount of protein, which helps the plant grow quickly. And the seeds have valuable minerals such as calcium, manganese, and phosphorus.

These are all nutrients that are unlikely to be found surrounding the seed when it lands in desert sands or soils and all particularly valuable. Again, because the chia seed is so small, it has to be packed with very concentrated amounts of these valuable nutrients, so that the especially tiny chia plant embryo inside the seed can get some momentum in trying to grow. This is what makes chia truly a "super" food.

The oils in chia seeds also have the side effect of creating a rich gel when the seeds are immersed in water, which slows digestion. This is a benefit that's uniquely valuable to modern humans.

How People Changed Chia

People have been cultivating all kinds of plants for at least thousands of years, if not much longer. We don't have detailed records for how this was done, but scientists have confirmed the basic outlines of how people tend to cultivate plants.

The basic trends are that people make the plant more convenient to grow and more productive in terms of the parts that people want to eat, but less hardy in nature—as plants that people are actively cultivating no longer have to compete in the wild.

The model for this approach is Gregor Mendel, the monk who began the modern science of genetics by carefully tracking experimental cross-breeding of peas in the mid-1800s. Mendel's work was a real breakthrough and later contributed to the pioneering work of Frances Crick and James Watson in discovering DNA.

However, before Mendel, no one we know of bred plants scientifically. People all over the world simply grew more of the plants that worked out well for them and ignored the plants that didn't.

FOOD FOR THOUGHT

Today, people have taken plant breeding to the extreme of actually genetically modifying plants. This potentially risky experiment on human health and the natural environment seems unnecessary when there are so many good foods, such as chia, that are under-researched and underused.

We can speculate that some of the desirable properties of chia may have been the result of "unnatural selection"—Native American farmers planting the seeds of plants that worked well for them and discarding the seeds of plants that didn't. This same process has been used all over the world to improve key crops such as wheat, rice, and maize.

Maize changed so much under cultivation that we can infer that Native Americans were sophisticated cultivators, and that this same expertise might have been applied to chia. However, advances by the Aztecs and others might have been lost when chia was suppressed between the arrival of the conquistadores and the rediscovery of chia just a few years ago.

Where Is Chia Grown?

Chia's native growing area is unknown, but Native Americans cultivated it from the U.S. Southwest, across Central America, and well down into South America. The name of the Mexican state of Chiapas means "chia river" or "chia water" in the Nahuatl language.

In the United States today, chia grows easily where it's hot at least a good part of the year—coastal and central California, southwestern Arizona, southern Texas and Louisiana, and all of Florida except the panhandle.

With a bit of work, chia can be grown other places, especially on the coast of the Pacific Northwest and in the dark, rich soil of the Southeast.

The Flavor of Chia

Chia seeds have a mild, nutty flavor. Any food or meal made with nuts is a natural place to add chia, and nuts are in all kinds of dishes, from cereals and breads to salads and meat dishes. Using chia instead of, or in addition to, the nuts in such recipes is a can't-miss way to use chia.

Using chia seeds directly on, or cooked into, your food is a bit limiting, though. Digesting chia is water intensive, so eating chia seeds can dry you out, absorbing moisture internally. This can result in constipation, especially if you don't normally drink a lot of water.

> **FOOD FOR THOUGHT**
> Chia absorbs up to 12 times its weight in water. So an ounce of chia—3 tablespoons—can absorb up to 12 ounces of water.

To avoid its drying properties, it's a good idea to consume much of your chia in a gel. You just combine $^1/_4$ cup chia seeds with $^3/_4$ cup water. After a couple of hours, the gel forms.

The gel tastes slightly earthy, as some red wines do. This isn't a problem, but the texture can be. It's a bit slimy, which can be offputting to some people.

Mixing chia gel in with the right foods makes a big difference. The texture just about disappears in yogurt, in a smoothie, or in granola. You'll need to try it yourself in other recipes to see what works for you and what doesn't.

The Least You Need to Know

- The chia plant is a bush that grows up to about 3 feet tall. The seeds are just 1 millimeter in diameter.
- Chia's high nutrition content is due in part to the harsh desert climate in which chia grows, as well as human cultivation.
- Chia seeds have a nutty flavor. When soaked in water or other liquid they form a gel.

Chia's Nutritional Profile

If you're interested in incorporating chia into your diet, it's important for you to understand why it's considered a superfood and how its unique nutritional profile can contribute to your overall health.

Chia is a superfood in five distinct ways:

1. As a source of fiber and as the creator of a gel that slows down digestion, both of which help manage diabetes

2. As an amazing source of omega-3 fatty acids, or "good fats," which work against heart disease

3. As a very efficient source of key minerals, including manganese, phosphorus, calcium, and iron

4. As an antioxidant with key compounds that are known to fight heart disease and certain cancers

5. As a long-lasting source of energy for endurance activities

These qualities make chia a great substitute for much of the meat and dairy in your diet, without many of the undesirable aspects of animal-based foods.

In This Chapter

- What makes chia a superfood
- How chia factors into your recommended daily allowances
- Chia's key nutrients and antioxidant properties
- Chia as a source of energy

With this knowledge at the ready, you can use chia seeds, other seeds, superfoods, and other healthy foods together for maximum benefit. We've touched on these topics before, but this chapter will take a closer look at the qualities that make the chia seed so special.

Superfoods versus Processed Foods

The whole idea behind adding superfoods to your diet is to eat foods that "punch above their weight." That is, a food that has more nutrients in it than most, making your whole diet more healthful.

The trouble is that we ask a lot of superfoods. Today's typical foods often have less nutrition than they once did, because they're grown in depleted soils. So if you were to make up your diet only from foods that were available, say, 100 years ago, you would probably get less nutrition from it than people of the time would have.

We also have a modern tendency that puts even more pressure on superfoods: the tendency to eat lots of processed and fast foods. Many processed and fast foods offer little in the way of nutrients or fiber. The "nutrients" they do have are often artificial or highly processed versions of known vitamins like vitamin A or vitamin D. This makes the foods look more nutritious, but they're still lacking less well-known or still undiscovered nutrients, and they are almost always lacking in healthy fiber.

Processed and fast food is also full of unhealthy fats, sugar, salt, and preservatives.

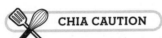 **CHIA CAUTION**

> You need fats, but healthy ones. You need sugar and salt, but you're likely to get them without trying. And you don't need preservatives.

Processed and fast foods are likely to contain GMOs (genetically modified organisms), which are not called out on food labels. And these types of foods are made from grains, fruits, and vegetables that are grown as monocultures in factory farms and from animals that are factory farmed as well.

The result is that much of what people in the developed world eat today is either lower in nutrients than we might expect (an apple, for instance, with perhaps 25 percent less nutrient value than an apple of 50 years ago) or filler with little food value (that is, processed food and fast food) and plenty of problematic stuff in it, too.

You almost have to eat lots of superfoods just to get back to a healthy diet!

Calories Count

Let's put some numbers around what we mean by foods that "punch above their weight." For important vitamins and minerals, the U.S. Department of Agriculture has assigned amounts you should eat each day. This is based on a 2,000 calorie diet for an adult. If you need more or fewer calories to maintain a healthy weight, you should scale up or down accordingly.

If you typically eat 2,000 calories per day, and you eat a breakfast that's 500 calories, you've eaten 25 percent of your daily value (DV) for calories. If your breakfast has 15 grams of fiber, that's about 50 percent of the recommended daily value. (The daily value for fiber varies with weight, age, and gender, like other DVs. Twenty-five grams is a guideline that you should adjust to your own needs.)

As we go through different categories of nutrition that chia seeds provide in the rest of this chapter, we'll compare what you get from chia to the recommended daily values. This is based on the following numbers:

- 1 serving chia = 3 tablespoons, 1 ounce, or 28 grams
- Recommended calories per day = 2,000 calories (adjust for your current and desired weight)
- Calories in 1 tablespoon of chia = 138, or 7 percent of your DV (daily value) for calories

If it's hard for you to think about calories in terms of percentages, try thinking of them as a fraction instead. In this case, 7 percent of your DV is equivalent to one fourteenth of your daily calorie intake.

The comparisons we provide here are just a starting point, but they'll give you a sense of what chia does for you—and where you need to use other foods to help build a healthy daily diet.

Recommended Daily Values

It's very valuable to understand and use the recommended daily amounts for different components of your diet. Use these numbers as guidelines and try to meet them.

The daily values don't include all the nutrients we need, and they certainly don't include the nutrients we don't understand well enough to measure yet. They also don't include special needs for people who are pregnant, growing up, exercising a lot, under stresses of various kinds, and so on.

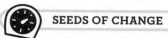 **SEEDS OF CHANGE**

> If you eat a diet with lots of fruits, vegetables, and healthy proteins, and one that meets the daily values for the known nutrients listed here, you're likely to also include most of the less-well-known nutrients for which we don't have daily value numbers.

Food Component	Daily Value (DV)	Chia 1 oz.*
Calories	2,000	138 (7%)
Total fat	65 grams (g)	8.6 grams (g) (13%)
Saturated fat	20 g	0.9 g (4%)
Cholesterol	300 milligrams (mg)	0
Total carbohydrate	300 g	12.3 g (4%)
Dietary fiber	25 g	10.6 g (42%)
Protein	50 g	5 g (10%)
Selected Minerals		
Manganese	2 mg	0.6 mg (30%)
Phosphorus	1,000 mg	265 mg (27%)
Calcium	1,000 mg	177 mg (18%)
Iron	18 mg	2.2 mg (13%)
Zinc	15 mg	1 mg (7%)
Copper	2 mg	0.1 mg (3%)
Potassium	3,500 mg	45 mg (1%)
Magnesium	400 mg	0
Sodium	2,400 mg	5 mg (0%)
Chloride	3,400 mg	0
Vitamins		
Vitamin A	5,000 International Units (IU)	0
Vitamin B_6	2 mg	0
Vitamin B_{12}	6 micrograms (μg)	0
Vitamin C	60 mg	0
Vitamin D	400 IU	0
Vitamin E	30 IU	0
Vitamin K	80 μg	0
Thiamin	1.5 mg	0
Riboflavin	1.7 mg	0
Niacin	20 mg	0
Folate	400 μg	0
Pantothenic acid	10 mg	0

Nutritional information for chia courtesy NutritionData.com

Fiber, Carbohydrates, and Sugar

Chia seeds are a wonderful source of fiber. Chia is a fiber "superfood." One ounce of chia has 10 grams of fiber. That's 40 percent of your daily fiber needs, in one small ounce. That ounce has a mere 7 percent of your daily calories. So chia has about five times more fiber than the average food in a balanced, nutritious diet.

Although it is high in fiber, one serving of chia has only 12 grams of carbohydrates—a mere 4 percent of the recommended total. Unlike the carbohydrates found in highly processed foods, which break down quickly during digestion and release sugar rapidly, those in chia break down slowly. This means chia is low on the *glycemic index*.

 DEFINITION

The **glycemic index** of a food measures the amount of sugar in a food and how quickly that sugar is absorbed in your system. For example, table sugar has a glycemic index of 100. Pairing high-glycemic-index foods with low-glycemic-index foods when you eat them "takes the edge" off the high-glycemic-index foods, reducing their effect on your system.

Chia is not only low in glycemic index; it forms a "gel" in your stomach that slows down the absorption of sugar. In effect, it lowers the glycemic index of everything else that you eat at the same time.

Many people who have, or want to avoid, diabetes are on the lookout for low-glycemic-index foods that have lots of nutrition. Chia more than fills the bill; it's a superstar for working against diabetes.

Good Fats

When people talk about "good fats," they're usually referring to unsaturated fats, in particular the omega-3 fatty acids. These unsaturated fats are thought to aid in the prevention of a variety of health issues, including cancer and heart disease. They are found in relatively few foods, most notably oily fish, such as salmon, albacore tuna, mackerel, and anchovies.

Chia is also a great source of omega-3s and is a good alternative for those who wish to naturally increase their intake of these beneficial fats without eating fish or fish oil.

Another family of unsaturated fats is the omega-6 fatty acids. Although these are more healthful than saturated fats, they have been linked to inflammation, a major risk factor for heart disease. Omega-6s are also found in many more foods than omega-3s.

People who eat carefully are constantly on the lookout for foods that are high in omega-3s and low in omega-6s. Beef, cheese, and milk are fairly strong here, but they must be pasture raised, not factory farmed like most meats and dairy, for the full effect. Even the best-raised beef and dairy are relatively high in fat and cholesterol.

Also, omega-3s make the journey into your body best if they're in foods that aren't cooked. In countries like the United States, where meats and fish are usually thoroughly cooked, it's harder to get the full omega-3 benefits of these ingredients.

For this reason, chia has an advantage. It boasts a rare three to one ratio of omega-3 fats to omega-6s and is most often eaten without cooking, so the omega-3s make it all the way into your body.

In addition to its great preponderance of omega-3s, chia is low in saturated fat and cholesterol free. It's a very desirable food indeed for anyone concerned about their heart health.

Antioxidant Goodness

Oxidation is any process by which oxygen helps break down chemical bonds, releasing energy. Fire is a fast oxidizing process, and it produces so much energy you can warm your hands or cook a roast by it. Rust is a slow oxidizing process.

Some oxidizing processes that take place within our bodies are like rust. Certain foods and metabolic processes combine to create an excess of "free radicals," compounds that float around in our bloodstream and help break down healthy molecules in a damaging way. It's like rusting from inside.

 FOOD FOR THOUGHT

Technically, a free radical is an atom or molecule that has an extra, unpaired electron in its outer shell. This is like a knob sticking out that tries to fit into any gap it can find in other atoms or molecules. When the free radical combines with the other atom or molecule, it can cause the other atom or molecule to break down, and then it moves on and do it all over again. This process is thought to contribute to aging and the beginning stages of cancer, not unrelated phenomena.

Free radicals can be tamed—made nonradical—by antioxidants. And chia is full of antioxidants. Some of the antioxidants in chia are quercetin, which fights fatigue as well as cancers, heart disease, and type 2 diabetes; chlorogenic acid, which fights cancer, diabetes, and heart disease; and caffeic acid, which is thought to fight colon cancer and heart disease.

Chia is even higher in antioxidants than blueberries, another superfood known for its antioxidant properties.

Unfortunately, science does not yet fully understand the slow, subtle biological processes that lead to heart disease and cancer. It's believed, however, that free radicals are a key factor—and that antioxidants help prevent both.

Great Source of Key Minerals

Chia has lots of several key minerals that are necessary for keeping your body in peak condition and can be hard to get otherwise:

- **Manganese (30 percent of Daily Value):** Manganese is good for strong bones and healthy connective tissues. Berries and fruits are other sources.

- **Phosphorus (27 percent of Daily Value):** Phosphorus is good for bones and connective tissues, as well as digestion and absorbing other nutrients. Meat and dairy are good sources of phosphorus, as are nuts and legumes.

- **Calcium (18 percent of Daily Value):** Calcium is best known food for its role in creating strong, healthy bones and teeth. It helps prevent colon cancer and guard against obesity. Sources include meat, dairy, nuts, and legumes.

- **Iron (13 percent of Daily Value):** Iron is a big component of blood, helping carry oxygen to your tissues. It's vital for growth and repair of many tissues and for metabolizing food. Sources include meat, legumes, lentils, and many vegetables.

As you can see, this list includes many key minerals that are most frequently found in meat and dairy. This allows chia to be used to replace some of the meat in your diet without any drop-off in these nutrients.

Long-Lasting Source of Energy

Chia is known as a long-lasting source of energy; this was perhaps its most prized value in Native American cultures, who valued it particularly for running and long journeys on foot.

It's said that a quantity of chia seeds roughly equal to a modern tablespoon could sustain a runner or traveler for a day. We're not in any way recommending that diet plan, but it is a good illustration for many of the other benefits of chia.

Chia forms a gel in your stomach that slows and moderates the digestion of foods. It has a fair number of calories for its weight—but those calories carry many key nutrients. It has "good fats" that contain energy of their own. It has key minerals, including minerals that help digestion.

Even for those of us who don't try to run from one side of Central America to the other on a pouch full of chia seeds, an endurance food can make a lot of sense. One of the difficulties in modern life is to balance our food and nutrient intake with our actual needs for energy and nutrition. A moderating factor like chia, plus all the good minerals and antioxidants, can help you take your focus off eating as a frequent activity and more as a supportive element to a healthy and balanced life.

Chia Is Gluten Free

One of the really marvelous things about chia seeds is that they can be used to make a healthy, wholesome gluten-free flour.

Gluten is a key component of wheat, barley, and some other grains. As the name suggests, it serves as a kind of glue, a connective matrix that survives and thrives in the high heat of, for instance, a pizza oven. Gluten provides much of the chewy "mouth feel" that we enjoy so much in breads and baked goods.

Unfortunately, gluten is known to cause problems for a small number of people and suspected of causing problems for others. It may cause an immune system response that isn't healthy for children and other living things. It's believed that some people are completely immune from any negative response to gluten, that some are wholly ill served by eating it, and that others should keep their gluten consumption low and balanced with other sources of food energy.

Historically, gluten has been a key component of the Western diet, but with growing awareness of gluten intolerance, there have been many efforts to provide gluten-free alternatives to pizza dough, bread dough, cookie dough, and so on. To someone raised on wheat and its many derivative products, these alternatives—based on, for instance, rice—tend to lack the flavor, consistency, and plain old yumminess of the originals.

Chia seed and flaxseed are two sources for baked goods that, when carefully used, taste an awful lot like the gluten-infused alternatives. Try the recipes in this book. You may be able to go largely or completely gluten-free much more easily than you expected.

The Least You Need to Know

- Chia is a great source of fiber, omega-3 fatty acids, and key minerals.
- Chia's antioxidant properties may help to prevent cancer.
- The nutrients in chia make it a long-lasting source of energy, ideal for endurance sports.
- Chia seeds can be used to make a gluten-free flour that is comparable to the flavor and texture of wheat flour in baked goods.

How Chia Can Help You Stay Healthy

In the previous chapter, we looked at the nutrients in chia and touched on their health benefits. This chapter more closely examines chia's nutritional properties to explain how they help you stay healthy.

There's just so much good in chia seeds. As you learn about what they can do for you and begin to integrate them into your life, you will see why they were valued so highly by Native American cultures.

It's worth thinking about life in earlier times to help grasp just how much difference chia can make in our own lives. Of course, ancient cultures didn't have our sophisticated measurement techniques for the components of foods. Instead, they were probably better than we are at listening to their bodies and at learning from experience.

It was also easier for our predecessors to do controlled experiments than it is for us—though they wouldn't have understood the term. In a village, food was seasonal, and variety was limited by what was available locally. There were no processed foods to confuse the issue. As foods went in and out of season or came into a village through trade, people could more easily track the effect of a specific food, like chia, against their diets.

In This Chapter

- How the fiber in chia can aid in digestion
- How chia can help to fight diabetes
- How the fatty acids in chia work to prevent heart disease
- The benefits of anti-oxidants and other key nutrients

Some people, at least, were also harder on their bodies than we are today. Warriors didn't have immense supply chains to provide them with sustenance before going into battle. Messengers had to carry most of their food with them.

In such an environment, the benefits of chia seeds would quickly become apparent—and they'd be felt in the person's body.

Don't just read the information in this chapter; use it as inspiration to try the many recipes in this book. Try to feel the effects in your body of the chia seed diet—and of everything that you eat and drink. You're likely to be healthier for it.

Chia as a Source of Fiber

Most people who add chia to their diet find that the effects of chia's high-fiber content are the most noticeable. This is a little sad, because it says as much about how poor our diets are, compared to what our bodies really need, as it does about how great chia is. While chia has many pronounced benefits, its ability to help address the West's severe deficit of fiber is perhaps its number one benefit.

Grains have only been a staple of the human diet for less than 10,000 years. In the millions of years of primate evolution before that, raw vegetables and grasses were the bulk of our diets. Fruits and meats came and went in the diet as they became available through seasonal changes and successful hunting.

In the last few thousand years, humans have begun eating more grain-rich diets and cooking more and more of our food. This has led to a decrease in our consumption of fiber. Modern inventions like white bread and white sugar are so low in fiber and digest so very quickly that they contribute to newly potent diseases such as diabetes and colon cancer. This latter disease is believed to be caused partly by "soft" diets that don't toughen up the colon; "soft" food accumulates, rots within the colon, and contributes to the beginnings of cancer cells.

If you eat a typical Western diet, you're highly likely to need more fiber. And what you need isn't light or weak or processed fiber, like you might find in "whole wheat" bread. You need the kind of fiber your body doesn't ever digest—insoluble fiber, like you find in "whole grain" bread.

This may seem counterintuitive, because "indigestible" sounds like something bad. But with fiber, it's very good. Insoluble, or indigestible, fiber takes up space in your stomach, slowing digestion, absorbing toxins from other food and drink. This beneficial "sponge" effect continues as the fiber passes through your intestines. The muscles that move food through your body actually get stronger as they have something to work against. And in the end (pun intended), you're much less likely to be constipated; your body is getting the kind of material it actually needs to keep your digestive tract working properly.

The following table shows key benefits of chia as a source of dietary fiber.

Key Benefits	Description
Daily intake	One ounce of chia has 11 grams of fiber, about 42 percent of the average recommended adequate intake.
Digestion barrier	All fiber slows digestion, but only chia forms a gel in the stomach that surrounds the food you eat, causing it to take longer to digest.
Effect on sugar	Chia, as a fiber and through the gel that it forms, slows the absorption of sugars in high glycemic index foods (such as table sugar or white bread).
Energy impact	More gradual digestion reduces feelings of "sugar high" and "sugar crash."
Dieting impact	All fiber makes you feel fuller longer, easing dieting. Chia's gel increases this effect.
Digestive impact	Fiber reduces constipation and bloating and cramping (unless overused). It also absorbs toxins from other food and drink.
Insoluble	About 85 percent of the fiber in chia is insoluble and therefore not digestible, which is a good thing. Chia slows digestion and exercises your intestines.
Equivalents	100 grams of chia is equivalent to nearly 300 grams of oats as a source of fiber.

 CHIA CAUTION

Take fiber recommendations with a grain of salt. Our ancestors ate far more fiber than we do, and we don't really know what's optimum for health. Also, fiber needs vary greatly with age and size. Increase your fiber intake gradually, and discuss diet changes with a healthcare professional.

Chia as a Diabetes Fighter

There are two main types of diabetes: type 1 and type 2. The two types affect the body in similar ways but are caused by different things. Type 1 diabetes is a hereditary disease caused by a single recessive gene. It affects children from shortly after birth.

Those with type 1 diabetes don't produce insulin and are therefore unable to process or store sugar in the same way as other people. To manage the disease, people with type 1 diabetes take insulin; this prevents sharp spikes in blood sugar. Paradoxically, they also need regular "injections" of sugary foods, such as fruit or even a donut, to keep their blood sugar from falling catastrophically low. (If blood sugar crashes in a person with type 1 diabetes, it can lead to a diabetic coma.)

Type 2 diabetes is different. It's more subtle. People with type 2 diabetes also have difficulty processing sugar, but they are not generally in danger of the same blood sugar spikes as type 1 diabetics, nor of a diabetic coma. Instead, the less-extreme swings in blood sugar of a type 2 diabetic cause gradual damage to cells—such as cells in the eyeball, leading to blindness—and to the linings of arteries. This not only causes heart attacks but other insidious problems such as poor circulation, leading to wounds that are slow to heal. More than 30,000 Americans have a foot amputated each year because type 2 diabetes has prevented wounds from healing.

Although the causes of type 2 diabetes are not completely understood, it is attributed to lifestyle factors as well as genetics. The lifestyle factors linked to type 2 diabetes include obesity, poor diet, and lack of exercise. Type 2 diabetes used to be called "adult onset diabetes" because it was normally only found in adults. However, in more recent years, the diet and exercise habits of many people have become so poor that "adult onset" diabetes is often seen in children.

As with fiber, chia is such a strong diabetes fighter partly because of weaknesses in current Western diets. Processed foods, which are new on the scene and still growing in their impact, are very high in sugar and easily soluble fibers that the body can convert to sugar almost instantly. (Eating a slice of white bread makes your blood sugar spike just as much as eating a spoonful of sugar.)

The fiber in chia and its tendency to form a gel that traps other foods both slow the absorption of whatever else you're eating. If that slice of white bread gets embedded in chia gel in your stomach, it's not going to create a burst of blood sugar in nearly the same way.

Diabetes is a disease caused by poor absorption of sugar from the blood. When the sugar isn't absorbed, it damages tissues it comes in contact with. In particular, it causes inflammation in vein and artery walls, contributing to the risk of stroke and heart attack. By helping sugar get absorbed, chia reduces this dangerous inflammation.

Chia also helps reduce blood pressure (systolic as well as diastolic), which just makes things easier on the stressed internal systems of diabetics.

Other complex compounds in chia, such as omega-3 fatty acids, also contribute to slower, more manageable digestion of all foods, including sugars and soluble fibers.

Due to poor diet and lack of exercise, many people in America today are *prediabetic*, or suffering from *metabolic syndrome*. We are overweight, our arteries are in trouble, our blood pressure is high—just less so than a typical diabetic. But being partway there increases our risk of diabetes and the problems associated with diabetes, even if we never cross the line into diabetes itself.

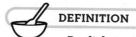

Prediabetes is when blood glucose levels are higher than normal but not yet high enough to be diagnosed as diabetes. Some people with prediabetes have symptoms of diabetes or even problems with diabetes already. **Metabolic disorder** is a combination of medical disorders that, when occurring together, increase the risk of developing cardiovascular disease and diabetes.

For these reasons, chia's diabetes-fighting qualities are valuable, even if you are not diabetic. Refer to the table in the previous section for benefits of chia as a diabetes fighter, as well as benefits as a source of fiber. The two kinds of benefits are inextricably linked.

Chia as a Source of Protein

Many people understand that protein is a vital part of one's diet, even more so for growing children. Protein helps create new muscle and repair all kinds of tissue.

Proteins are made up of different amino acids. The human body makes some and depends on the food you eat for others. For the most part, you have to eat foods balanced in the "missing" amino acids all at the same time. That way, the body can combine the needed proteins and the ones your body makes to form a complete protein and put that to work in your body.

If some amino acids are missing, no complete proteins are formed; the "extra" amino acids are just burned by your muscles for (quite powerful) fuel. Unfortunately for vegetarians and vegans, plant-based foods tend to contain only some of the needed amino acids; they have to be combined with complementary foods, or the person eating them misses out on complete proteins. Meat, fish, and eggs, however, do have complete proteins.

Chia seeds are really unusual for plants in that they have complete proteins. Most seeds and nuts share this distinction, because they are the starting food for young plants, which need complete proteins, too. But chia seeds are also extremely versatile—they're easy to add to almost any meal with little noticeable flavor or texture.

People who go vegetarian or vegan often worry about getting complete protein in their diet. Chia is an excellent part of the solution.

Chia and Heart Disease

Chia can also be an effective tool in the prevention of heart disease. Many of the nutrients in chia have been shown to reduce blood pressure, inflammation, and cardiovascular problems—all of which contribute to the risk of heart attack.

Major concerns for those watching their heart health include the damaging effects of meat and dairy. Chia does a lot to replace meat and dairy in the diet or to augment modest amounts of meat and dairy while providing many nutrients that would otherwise go missing.

Meat and dairy are also among the most satisfying foods in staving off hunger in those trying to balance their diets. Chia is effective this way as well. So chia can, again, take up much of the weight of meat and dairy without the resulting problems.

The Benefits of Chia's Omega-3s

If you recall from Chapter 3, we mentioned chia is full of heart-healthy omega-3 fatty acids. We've been trained to think of fats as bad, but the truth is that our bodies need fats to work properly, and fatty acids are part of that. As we discussed in Chapter 3, there are two main types of fatty acids: omega-3 fatty acids and omega-6 fatty acids. For optimal heart and artery health, you should take in a certain amount of fatty acids, in a balance of roughly three to one in favor of omega-3s.

Omega-3s and omega-6s in this balance lower your blood pressure; reduce the risk of arthritis; help prevent cardiac arrhythmia, a leading contributor to heart attacks; and reduce the incidence of depression.

Unfortunately, omega-3s are relatively rare in most of our food sources. That's because our food sources today have moved a long way from what we evolved to need. Steak and other beef tends to have far more omega-6 fatty acids than omega-3s. A modern diet can easily have 10 times more omega-6 fatty acids than omega-3s.

 FOOD FOR THOUGHT

Grass-fed beef has a nearly healthy balance of fatty acids, but the more common feedlot-raised beef is higher in omega-6s.

The most easily accessible foods that are rich in omega-3s almost all have problems for the average consumer:

Salmon: Salmon is rich in omega-3s, especially raw salmon—as found in sushi. But salmon has a fairly strong flavor that not everyone likes, and it can be quite expensive, especially when delivered as sushi.

Solid albacore tuna: Wild-caught, unprocessed albacore tuna is rich in omega-3s. It's also the most expensive kind of tuna. As with salmon, eating albacore tuna raw, as sushi, is especially beneficial and especially expensive.

Mackerel: Mackerel is a very strong-flavored fish that is packed with omega-3s, too. Mackerel is not nearly as expensive as salmon or tuna, so if you are among those who like the flavor, eat it.

Chia: Chia is not very expensive, does not have any kind of fishy flavor, and is easy to eat raw. The only problem with chia is working reasonable amounts of it into your diet, as this book demonstrates throughout.

As with fiber, chia stands out as a superfood partly because of regrettable deficiencies in our modern diet. Among the natural, wild foods people ate before agriculture, omega-3s were abundant—and our bodies evolved to adapt to this balance. But as agriculture, domestication of animals for meat, and cooking and processing of food took hold, omega-6 fatty acids became more prevalent. The generally positive things we are doing to control our food supply for more reliability and variety have also degraded that same food supply in important ways.

One way to offset this is to augment our food chain. In a 1995 study, chickens were fed chia seeds. Their eggs featured increased omega-3 levels, with no off-flavor. You may be able to buy such eggs in your area or to "grow" your own if you raise chickens yourself.

The following summarizes the benefits of the omega-3 fatty acids found in chia.

Key Benefits	Description
Daily intake	One ounce of chia seeds represents more than 100 percent of recommended omega-3 fatty acid intake. Significantly offsets abundance of omega-6s in average diet.
Omega-3 source	Chia is one of the best food sources of omega-3s.
Dieting impact	Much less need for grass-fed beef and wild fish to get benefits of omega-3s.
Equivalents	Once ounce of chia seeds has same amount of omega-3s as 8 ounces of salmon.

Antioxidant Benefits of Chia

Chia is full of antioxidants. They are there for a simple reason. Chia seeds are rich in oil and fat to feed the fledgling chia plant. The antioxidants prevent these oils from breaking down before the plant embryo needs them. The antioxidants in chia have the same beneficial effects in your bloodstream.

Technically, antioxidants are chemicals with OH combinations sticking out of a longer molecule. The OH combination is an oxygen atom and a hydrogen atom. Other foods that you eat contain "free radicals"—compounds with a single oxygen atom sticking out, ready to cause trouble by combining with otherwise stable compounds that your body needs. Toxins tend to generate free radicals in your body.

> **FOOD FOR THOUGHT**
>
> Lead is an example of a toxin that generates free radicals. Other heavy metals do the same thing. Extra electrons in heavy metals transfer to other atoms and molecules, making them free radicals. And lead and other heavy metals interact with oxygen to produce a highly radical form of oxygen.

Antioxidants work in different ways to disrupt the progress of damaging reactions caused by free radicals. You actually need a rich mix of antioxidants to combat the damaging effects of everything from ultraviolet radiation to pesticides.

Chia has several of the major antioxidants, but it is not a substitute for other sources of antioxidant compounds, such as fruit. Instead, it's a key component in your antioxidant arsenal. If you see one antioxidant food compared to another, the measurement tells you something about relative potency, but the effects of antioxidants are cumulative—much like, unfortunately, the effects of free radicals. Don't trade off the effects of one antioxidant-rich food for another; avoid toxins, such as pesticides, and cultivate multiple sources of antioxidants in your diet.

The following table summarizes the benefits of the antioxidants found in chia.

Key Benefits	Description
Variety of antioxidants	Chia has useful amounts of chlorogenic acid, caffeic acid, kaemforol, myricetin, quercetin, and other antioxidants known as flavonols.
Bone health	Antioxidants help preserve bone mass, which can otherwise deteriorate under assault from free radicals. They complement the role of calcium in saving bone mass.
Equivalents	Chia is similar to blueberries, a very powerful source of antioxidants, on a gram for gram basis—and nine times as potent as oranges.
Sources	Sprouted chia flour is an even stronger source of antioxidants than chia seeds or regular chia flour.

Additional Benefits of Chia

We've already discussed chia as a great source of fiber and omega-3 fatty acids, as a combatant against diabetes, and as a source of antioxidants. Chia is also a great source for some of the vitamins and minerals your body needs to stay healthy.

Calcium: On an ounce for ounce basis, chia has six times the calcium of whole milk. Calcium is needed for building and repairing bodily tissues, such as bones. So if you have an ounce of chia seeds and a 6-ounce glass of whole milk, you get a significant portion of the calcium you might need in a day.

Iron: Chia has four times the iron of spinach on an ounce for ounce basis. Iron helps carry oxygen in your blood, so you need a steady supply. If you eat lots of red meat, you get lots of iron, and lots of not so good stuff, too. Chia gives you the iron without the headaches. (In fact, it mitigates problems from the meat you do consume.)

Vitamin C: An ounce of chia has as much vitamin C as several oranges, long famous as the main food source for vitamin C. Vitamin C is a powerful antioxidant.

Magnesium: Chia has roughly twice as much magnesium, ounce for ounce, as a nut such as walnuts. Magnesium is needed for generating energy from food and for sexual functioning for both genders.

Potassium: Chia also has about twice as much potassium, per ounce, as a banana. Potassium is also needed for generating energy and sexual functioning.

As you can see, chia is a nutritional powerhouse and a wonderful tool for those who wish to address the deficits left by the modern diet.

The Least You Need to Know

- Chia is high in fiber, with three times the fiber of oats per gram, and helps you feel full longer.
- Chia helps your body process food energy gradually, which is beneficial to those with diabetes or metabolic syndrome.
- Chia is full of heart-healthy fatty acids, particularly omega-3s. Per ounce, it has eight times more omega-3s than salmon.
- The antioxidants in chia help your body fight cancer-causing free radicals.
- Chia is rich in vitamins and minerals, including calcium, iron, and vitamin C.

Bringing Chia into Your Life

Now that you know how chia can benefit you, it's time to learn how to get it into your daily life. This part includes discussion of how strong a complement chia is to existing diets, such as vegan and vegetarian, gluten-free, low-carb, and paleo.

You also learn about other products with chia you can buy, such as premade chia foods and even personal-care products. You then get a shopping list for the foods and ingredients you should have on hand when beginning this chia seed diet journey.

Chia with Other Diets

Chia is a great kick starter for quick weight loss and can "prime the pump" for moving to a healthier diet overall. Its many advantages can make a real and sudden difference in your health.

But no single food—even a super superfood like chia—can meet all, or nearly all, your dietary needs. Also, the mainstream Western diet has so many unhealthy aspects—and so many nutritional gaps—that not even chia can replace all the bad stuff and fill in all of the holes where good stuff should be.

In this chapter, we'll describe several popular diet alternatives that you can consider, or even that you may already be following, and how chia can help augment them. With chia, you can help make the diet not only adequate but truly positive for your daily and long-term health.

In This Chapter

- Chia with vegan and vegetarian diets
- Chia with gluten-free diets
- Chia with low-carb diets
- Chia with paleo diets

How Diets Developed

Ever since humans evolved as a separate group of species a few million years ago, all of humanity has been involved in an evolutionary process that's competitive and cooperative with existing plants and animals and with other humans. Successful cultures get several things right in order to survive and prosper. One of the things they get right is food.

A culture that develops a nutritious cuisine that's complete, adaptable to the seasons, easy enough to prepare, and healthy enough to sustain a population with relatively little disease is far more likely to prosper. Within the overall culture, different habits and practices relating to food make specific groups healthier, happier, and more successful. It's far from a perfect process, but it's a workable one—cultures compete among internal groups and with other cultures, and the cultures that are more successful grow and thrive. Less-successful cultures tend to wither away and get absorbed—gradually or forcibly—by neighboring groups.

Different cultures each developed a "package" of core foods that met the needs for calories, proteins, vitamins, minerals, and fiber. The package had to work year-round, taking into account seasonality and the lack of refrigeration faced by nearly all cultures. (In some environments, a culture has access to cool or cold places for food storage year-round, or nearly so; in other environments, not so much.)

This package of core foods evolved over centuries and millennia, and dietary habits, daily routines that incorporated more or less exercise, and various folkways (or habits) evolved dealing with food availability and food choices.

 FOOD FOR THOUGHT

> Drinking too much alcohol can certainly lead to health problems. But used properly, wine can be worth its weight in, well, wine is a good example, as it's pretty darn valuable by the ounce.
>
> For instance, red wine contains antioxidants. French people eat lots of butter, which has fats that can damage the arteries. But the antioxidants in red wine combat this tendency. It turns out that, if you're going to use a lot of butter in your cooking, having a reasonable amount of red wine with your meal can be a good thing. So the French folkway of having a small glass of red wine with lunch may turn out to be a very good thing indeed for many French people.

For instance, in the book *French Women Don't Get Fat,* author Mireille Guiliano points out that French women don't, well, get fat, nor do French people tend to develop heart disease, despite eating what seems to be amazing amounts of butter and foods prepared in butter and drinking quite a bit of wine to boot. She explains that the overall French diet, work habits, play habits—the entire culture, including food—have had thousands of years to evolve in a healthy and sustainable direction. French people have habits, many of which they may never think about consciously, that make having some dishes with lots of butter quite tolerable in the big picture of how French people eat, drink, and live.

Both agriculture and urbanization put a lot of pressure on a culture's food resources, because they encourage strong growth in populations, but only if people can be fed adequately. This was especially difficult before recent years, when refrigeration became commonly available. Urban people don't have ready access to farm or forest (or jungle), so foraging and access to fresh food of any type are very limited.

As populations exploded in Europe, urbanization increased, and feeding people became a real problem. Without refrigeration, storing food was as big a problem as any—and storing meat, the most efficient source of complete protein, was a problem all its own.

For example, the French and the British can be seen as developing rival solutions to this problem. The French are said to have developed delicious, sophisticated sauces so as to cover up the taste of "high," gamy, or even rancid meat. The British, on the other hand, are said to simply boil everything in water to an extreme degree—pardon my pun—especially meats. Boiling produced a far more bland diet that didn't try to hide the substance of what was in food or what was left in the food after all that boiling.

You can play this same game with cultures and cuisines that you're familiar with. Every culture faced problems with food relating to seasonal availability of different foods, access to refrigeration (both cool and truly cold), nutrition, freshness, and attractiveness of the resulting cuisine. And every culture solved those problems in different ways.

Until the last few hundred years, most people around the world lived close to where they were born and to where their parents were born as well. They lived in cultures that had adapted to a locality over centuries or millennia. Whatever cuisine they ate, it had to have stood the test of time, by definition. The cuisine and other elements of culture co-evolved to create a workable whole.

Vegetarian and Vegan Diets

A vegetarian diet can be considered a sacrifice for some people, yet it allows everything you need for a complete, healthy diet. In fact, the definition of a vegetarian diet is so broad that it's quite possible to eat a very unhealthy diet—even a McDonald's-centric diet with French fries, Filet of Fishes, and large sodas—while staying more or less vegetarian.

FOOD FOR THOUGHT

One of our authors once heard a yoga teacher describe himself as a "phylo-genetic elitist." He included chicken in his "vegetarian" diet, on the theory that avoiding eating mammals—that is, beef, pork, lamb, horsemeat, and other such meats—qualified him as a type of vegetarian.

Vegetarians eat fruit, vegetables, nuts, seeds, eggs, dairy products, and sometimes fish (vegetarians who eat fish are called *pescatarians*). There's often a moral basis for various forms of vegetarianism; cattle and pigs, for instance, can be seen as higher animals, making causing them pain and premature death something people following vegetarianism don't condone.

Related to a moral basis for vegetarianism, some religions, such as many Hindu sects, ban or restrict the eating of meat. Observant Muslims and Jews follow dietary proscriptions—halal for Muslims, kosher for Jews—that ban some foods, such as pork, and give specific ways to prepare others, especially meats that aren't banned altogether.

Many vegetarians, understanding just how easy it is for their diet to be corrupted with processed and unhealthy foods, also watch what they eat closely in other ways. One of the ways is by following the raw food movement. Raw foods devotees eat mostly or entirely foods that are not only not processed, but not cooked. They don't eat anything, or much of anything, that your many-greats grandmother wouldn't recognize as food: no breads or anything canned, frozen, puréed, or otherwise altered from the way it comes out of the ground or off of a tree.

Vegan diets are more limited. A vegan diet is what someone who didn't know the word might think a vegetarian diet meant: a vegetable-based diet with fruit, nuts, and grains, but no meat, eggs, dairy, or fish. Everything from the plant kingdom, nothing from the animal kingdom.

Potential Obstacles in Vegetarian and Vegan Diets

The main problem with vegetarian and, especially, vegan diets is the paucity of protein. A mainstream Western diet features way too much meat, given that meat tends to be fatty and contain lots of antibiotics and other chemicals due to the way livestock is raised in Western countries. However, all that meat makes it very likely indeed that your needs for complete proteins are met.

FOOD FOR THOUGHT

More recently, additional reasons for "going veg" have emerged. Raising animals for any purpose, especially to eat them as food, generates lots of greenhouse gas emissions. And mainstream animal husbandry is increasingly likely to involve animals standing in their own feces for weeks and months in feedlots or crowded pens, raising the specter of serious health problems for the animals and anyone who eats them.

Having no meat at all—and no eggs, in a fully vegan diet—means you have a challenge getting enough protein. There are other needed elements, such as iron and vitamin B_{12}, that also tend to be found in abundance in meat and not in great quantities anywhere else.

Given the problems with meat, especially factory-farmed beef, a fully vegan diet with lots of raw foods is probably healthier than a mainstream diet, even if it leaves you a bit weak and anemic. While many people are vegan on most meals, rather than all the time, this isn't an option for strict vegetarians, including people operating under moral or religious regimes.

If you "go veg"—switch to a mostly or entirely vegetarian or vegan diet—you'll be looking for other sources of protein, as well as other now-missing nutrients, such as iron and B_{12}.

How Chia Can Supplement Vegetarian and Vegan Diets

Luckily, chia provides many of the pieces that are likely to be hard to come by in a vegetarian or vegan diet:

- **Healthy fats:** Chia is one of the few fat sources that has a healthy balance of omega-3 and omega-6 fatty acids.

- **Iron:** One ounce of chia has about one eighth (13 percent) of your daily iron requirement.

- **Other minerals:** An ounce of chia has about a third of your daily needs for manganese and phosphorus (the latter of which is mostly provided to us by meat) and a fifth of your need for calcium (otherwise largely found in milk and cheese).

Chia can even be used to substitute for eggs, allowing you to make healthy dishes that directly replace some of the more tempting offerings that you may indulge yourself in if you're not vegan.

Chia also helps solve two of the key issues faced by vegans and vegetarians. The first is feeling hungry. Part of this problem is path dependent: People who are used to the concentrated punch of calories and fat found in a steak or a cheeseburger are likely to feel hungry even when they're actually full, simply because they're accustomed to the very dense impact of meat. This impact tends to fade over time as vegetarians and vegans get used to the absence (or, in some cases, near-absence) of meat in their diets. But part of feeling hungry as a vegetarian or vegan is more genuine; our ancestors ate a lot more than we did to feel full because they were eating less-dense food. To eat enough to feel full on a vegetarian diet, you're likely to spend a lot of time preparing food and eating, and you're likely to take in more calories than you actually need for today's largely sedentary lifestyles.

The second issue is a sudden drop-off in energy. You can also be subject to blood sugar crashes as more easily digested foods, lacking the staying power of meat, pass through your system more quickly. Again, you either spend a fair amount of time eating and preparing food or a fair amount of time feeling hungry.

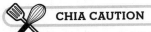   **CHIA CAUTION**

One ounce of chia has more than 4 grams of protein, while your daily need for protein is roughly a number of grams equal to a third of your body weight (in pounds). So if you're a moderately active man of 200 pounds, you need about 70 grams of protein a day. Even if you're a slip of a thing at 100 pounds, you need about 35 grams of protein a day. That's a lot of chia!

So rather than depending on chia, look to other foods compatible with a vegetarian or vegan diet, such as beans (especially the traditional Aztec/Mexican combination of beans and corn), tofu or other soy products, and quinoa.

Chia can help you with these issues by making you feel full and helping your body extract energy from food more gradually. This makes meals more satisfying and keeps a high baseline of energy in your system for longer.

With all its goodness, chia is also free from many of the issues that can arise when you start eating lots and lots of plant-based food to make up for the absence of meat. For instance, chia is gluten free (see the next section), so it's not adding to problems you might have digesting foods made from wheat. There's just about nothing negative to worry about when you use chia to help augment and extend your vegan or vegetarian diet.

Gluten-Free Diets

One of the biggest mysteries—and one of the biggest sources of problems for people in their diet—is the presence of gluten in grains, such as barley, rye, and especially wheat. Unfortunately, the exact extent of the problems caused by gluten is part of what's mysterious. Why is this?

As we described earlier in this chapter, people evolved to eat certain foodstuffs that were prevalent in the environment where they lived. The way foodstuffs were identified as such, selected for use in the diet, and processed or not processed before eating are all cultural factors that evolve over many years, even thousands or tens of thousands of years. The time period over which this cultural evolution takes place is so long, it's often found to be accompanied by biological evolution as well. This is likely the case with wheat and wheat gluten, or gluten.

People only started eating a lot of wheat after the last Ice Age ended about 12,000 years ago. As people settled more into agricultural communities, wheat was a very tempting crop opportunity in the Middle East and across Europe. In fact, it became the single most important foodstuff in these regions in general, matched by corn in the Americas and rice in Asia.

All of these core foodstuffs could be cultivated more or less intensively and support much larger populations of people who were far less likely to starve during the winter, especially a particularly long or intense winter. Of course, being so dependent on one crop also increased the likelihood of malnutrition; if rice, for instance, is the only thing available at the end of that hard winter, you're going to be malnourished. But at least you'll be alive.

There's a problem specific to wheat and people with a lot of wheat in their food environment: Not everyone can digest wheat gluten well. In fact, some people can't digest it at all. One of the biggest quandaries people find themselves in as they try to create a healthy diet is the mystery of wheat gluten.

An estimated 1 or 2 percent of the population in the United States have celiac disease. People with celiac disease can't process wheat gluten at all, and eating wheat causes them serious health problems.

Most people with celiac disease are undiagnosed or misdiagnosed. Therefore, there are a lot of people out there who have celiac disease and don't know it. Symptoms of celiac disease include the following:

- Bloating
- Gas
- Diarrhea
- Fatigue
- Headaches
- Infertility
- Discolored teeth

When celiac disease is left untreated, it can lead to the development of other autoimmune diseases, osteoporosis, thyroid disease, and cancer.

There is also some portion of the population that doesn't have celiac disease but is gluten intolerant. No one knows exactly what gluten intolerance is nor how many people have it, and to what degree. Part of the confusion over gluten intolerance stems from the fact that gluten is extremely useful stuff.

Processed foods often have wheat gluten added to give them body and cohesion. Gluten doesn't show up on the list of ingredients on packaged foods, and many products with gluten in them—for natural reasons, or because it's been added—are sold without labels, such as bread or cakes in a bakery.

As Western culture has spread out to influence the whole world, and as movement and migration between regions have accelerated, gluten exposure is increasing everywhere. For making Western-style foods, gluten is so useful that avoiding it is difficult, and avoiding it completely is nearly impossible, unless you go on a diet that may seem pretty darn extreme.

Another part of the problem with understanding gluten intolerance comes from the fact that it's hard to diagnose it (unlike celiac disease, which is more severe and therefore easier to diagnose). It's a trial-and-error process that requires avoiding all of the many foods with gluten in them. And there's a lot of error in the trial; people don't always know that gluten is in a given food, and they often give into temptation and eat known gluten-containing foods anyway. (If you hear the words "Happy Birthday to you" being sung in your office, you can be pretty darn sure you're about to be tempted with some gluten-rich foods.)

 CHIA CAUTION

One problem with diagnosing gluten intolerance that we believe is severely underrated is that people haven't had time to adapt, culturally or biologically, to the onslaught of processed foods that have appeared over the last few thousand years. This includes the explosion in popularity over the last couple of centuries and the last few decades, as canning, packaged foods, and refrigeration all became far more common.

Potential Obstacles in Gluten-Free Diets

People can go on a gluten-free diet either as an experiment to try to determine if they're gluten intolerant or as a lifestyle choice because they believe they are or might be gluten intolerant. The nice thing for these people's health—but the confusing thing for understanding gluten intolerance—is that going gluten free also means avoiding whole swathes of processed foods, baked goods, and other stuff that was not considered food, or just not available, until very recently in evolutionary terms.

If the substitutes that people take on for all this stuff are even somewhat healthy, those people in question are going to get healthier. They're going to experience improvement in their bloating, gas, diarrhea, fatigue, headaches, infertility, or discolored teeth. They may well lose weight, feel better, and have their sex life pick up.

But we don't know for sure if the improvement comes from a better diet, from avoiding problematic substances found in all processed foods, such as preservatives, or from avoiding gluten specifically. So the great mass experiment that's going on with the spread of gluten-free alternative foods isn't telling us all that much about the actual prevalence and intensity of true gluten intolerance.

However, for people who don't have celiac disease or very strong gluten intolerance, it might not matter much. Avoiding foods with gluten is going to mean avoiding processed foods. With just a bit of care, it will also mean eating more raw and less-processed foods. So you're likely to get healthier but not necessarily know whether it's from eating less gluten or because of a better diet overall.

How Chia Can Supplement Gluten-Free Diets

Here's where chia comes in. Chia flour can be used to make all of the same foods as wheat flour. It's not an exact substitute; chia flour acts more like whole wheat flour than like processed wheat flour, so it's somewhat harder to cook with, and the results are grainier than with processed wheat flour. Luckily, more people are becoming aware of the benefits of whole-wheat flour anyway, so goods made with chia flour are not going to seem as strange as they would have just a few years ago.

Chia flour is also much more nutritious than regular wheat flour (which has little food value and almost no fiber) or whole-wheat flour (which is a little better).

Baked goods tend to punch way below their weight in terms of nutrition versus calories, especially if icings or other sweet flavorings are added on top or in the dish. Baked goods made with chia are better, but still not as good as, say, raw foods. So consider using chia as a substitute for wheat flour when you really need to, say, make a birthday cake, but shifting away from baked goods of any type to a great extent as you move away from gluten and processed foods and toward a healthier diet.

Chia with Low-Carb Diets

Carbohydrates are foods that are made up of lots of molecules that include carbon and water. Carbohydrates tend to generate a lot of energy in your body. Simpler carbohydrate molecules, such as sugars, are digested very quickly by your body. But highly processed flours, such as bleached white flour, are processed just as quickly. These fast-digesting foods give you a sugar rush in your bloodstream and then are quickly processed. The sudden sugar surge actually strains your system, and an hour later, all the food value is gone—you're hungry again. This has led to people going to low-carb diets, with the two most well-known being the Atkins diet and the South Beach diet.

 FOOD FOR THOUGHT

For a dramatic rendition of what happens when you eat sugar, see *The Atkins Diet* book; for a more moderate description, *The South Beach Diet* is a good source.

Potential Obstacles in Low-Carb Diets

Low-carb diets dramatically reduce the number of carbs you eat, especially simpler carbs. For example, people are not allowed to eat bread at all, at first, and only high-fiber breads later. Fruit juice is banned or strictly limited, because sugar in liquid is the easiest thing of all for your body to absorb. Alcoholic drinks are banned early and then restricted later, for the same reason. (Beer is not sweet at all, but it's metabolized very quickly, as is white wine; red wine is digested much more slowly.) Even fruit is banned from the early stages of many low-carb diets and restricted in the later stages, because while the pulp of the fruit does slow the digestion of sugars, there's still quite a punch in there.

Sodas are completely banned from all low-carb diets—even diet sodas, which ironically seem to trigger the same cycle of sugar rush and sudden hunger as sodas that actually have sugar in them. Pasta and potatoes also aren't allowed and are replaced by nothing (for pasta), and yams (for potatoes). And pizza, being basically bread, is not part of the diet either.

Low-carb diets have many of the benefits of other diets described in this chapter. They tend to move you away from processed foods, which tend to be full of sugar and carbs, and toward healthier choices such as raw foods. But low-carb diets do tend to be heavy in meat and even fat. For example, the Atkins diet is meat heavy and fat heavy by design (and proud of it), while the South Beach diet features less emphasis on meat and fat but can still lead people to a lot of meat because they've cut so many other foods out of their diet.

It's also possible to move to a low-carb diet and not get much healthier. There are more and more processed foods out there with lots of hidden calories, unhealthy fats, and preservatives that still earn the low-carb imprimatur.

How Chia Can Supplement Low-Carb Diets

Chia has fatty acids that you can usually get from meat, plus a preponderance of beneficial omega-3 fatty acids over omega-6s. The gel chia forms in your stomach is filling, which helps reduce cravings for all those donuts you're not eating and fruit juices and alcoholic drinks you're not drinking on a low-carb diet.

Because low-carb diets are subtraction diets—even the name says so—another great feature of chia comes to the forefront. Chia is easily made into flour that substitutes for whole-wheat flour while being even richer in fiber and nutrients. This allows you to make baked goods that substitute chia flour for wheat flours and stay on the less-restrictive later stages of most low-carb diets.

If you think of your low-carb diet as strictly taking things away, you're more likely to stay with many of your unhealthy habits. But if you think of the diet as an opportunity to move to healthier foods and take time to enjoy the new things that you can move to—such as raw foods, unprocessed foods, and chia—you're more likely to have a significantly healthier lifestyle and better results.

Chia and Paleo Diets

The paleo diet is a strict application of some of the ideas we've mentioned throughout this book. Paleo is short for Paleolithic, which refers to the Stone Age, or the time from the earliest recognizable humans a couple of million years ago to a period roughly 10,000 years ago when the last Ice Age ended and people started working with metals—leading to the Bronze Age and the Iron Age, then into modern culture.

Paleo diets harken back to the time when humans had not yet developed agriculture. We evolved for most of our evolutionary history without agriculture, so there's solid logic to this. Paleo diets include prehistoric foods such as wild greens, fruits in season, nuts, and meat; they exclude large quantities of grains and any kind of processed foods.

Potential Obstacles in Paleo Diets

The paleo diet takes all its foods from preagricultural times. Meats, vegetables, and fruits are the main foods consumed on this diet. Nuts are a natural candidate, but they—along with chia—are controversial in the paleo community.

Strictly speaking, chia does not fit into a paleo diet, because it contains phytic acid—an acid that's said to bind with minerals and take them out of your body, where they're useless to your body. Nuts also contain lots of phytic acid, yet they were of course common food for our ancestors (and their predecessors, who were apes) all over the world. In fact, cracking nuts, processing them into meal, and storing them are part of the technological development that made us fully human.

Phytic acid has also been shown to have beneficial effects as an antioxidant and cholesterol fighter. So paleo diet adherents argue energetically about phytic acid in general and specific foods—such as various types of nuts, which have differing phytic acid profiles, and chia—in particular.

How Chia Can Supplement Paleo Diets

Our opinion is that the ideas behind paleo diets are very attractive, but that a paleo diet is quite restrictive and very hard to follow. Within a general construct of all things in moderation, it's hard to see the sense of keeping either nuts or chia out of a paleo-only or paleo-mostly diet.

With this caveat, chia is very helpful for those who are on a fully or mostly paleo diet. As with other diets, chia fills a big gap in terms of helping you feel full when you might otherwise be thinking about all the different foods you're not eating. It provides a healthy source of fiber and a way to make "bridge" foods—such as occasional baked goods—that fill in the gap left by mainstream breads and so on, but with lots of fiber and nutrition and without the diabetes-inducing blood sugar spike caused by many such foods.

The Least You Need to Know

- Diets are created over thousands of years based on how different cultures adapt to what's available and what's not in their environment.
- Chia provides fatty acids missing from vegan and vegetarian diets, in a healthy preponderance of omega-3s.
- Chia flour is a gluten-free and low-carb flour that substitutes well for whole-wheat flour in those diets.
- Chia, like nuts, has phytic acid, making it controversial in paleo diets.

Getting Chia into Your Diet

As you learned in the previous chapter, chia is not only a strong addition to mainstream diets, it's a vital building block for comfortably moving to alternative diets that can do an awful lot for your health, including vegetarian and vegan diets, low-carb diets, gluten-free diets, and paleo diets.

But *how* do you use chia in your cooking? This chapter gives you the rundown of the different ways to prepare and use chia and the optimal level of chia you should consume daily.

In This Chapter

- Ways you can use chia
- Chia seeds and gels
- Chia as a replacement for refined flour and eggs
- Your optimal chia intake

How to Use Chia

There are five basic ways to use chia:

1. Directly as a seed, added to food just before you eat it or during cooking.

2. Mixed with water and refrigerated to form a gel that you add to foods just before you eat them.

3. As an egg substitute that you cook into foods to replace the consistency—and some of the nutrition—of eggs.

4. As a flour for coating foods before you fry them and for baking.

5. Embedded in prepared foods (see Chapter 7).

The first four require some planning and preparation on your part, so let's go through each of them in depth.

 FOOD FOR THOUGHT

You can get chia as white seeds, black seeds, or a mix. Black chia seeds come from the long, extended purple flowers on a chia plant, while white chia seeds come from the small white flowers. Which should you buy? Either or both is the short answer.

Experts say black seeds have a bit more antioxidants, while white seeds have a touch more protein. However, there can also be variation across plants and across growing seasons, so the difference between white and black seeds is quite minor.

If you have a choice, we suggest a mix of white and black seeds, just so you can be sure you're not missing anything.

Using Chia as a Seed

Chia seeds are a great way to get more water in your diet. They absorb water at a proportion of approximately 10 to 1. There are 48 teaspoons in a cup, so for every teaspoon of chia, drink an extra 10 teaspoons of water—a little less than 2 ounces. This will put you ahead in beneficial water consumption.

Including chia seeds in your meal also lowers the effective glycemic index of food. This means foods that would normally be digested very quickly, triggering a quick release of insulin and leaving you feeling tired, are digested more slowly. You feel full longer and can eat less without feeling hungry.

Uncooked chia seeds hardly have any taste at all, so you can add them to foods without noticing a significant difference. Plus, the seeds are so small, they don't cause any problems with chewing your food. There are 3 teaspoons in a tablespoon, so carry that amount of chia seeds with you in a plastic zipper-lock bag or small container, and try to sprinkle a spoonful on almost everything you eat. If you do this with every meal, you'll have your first tablespoon of chia for the day.

The following are a few examples of ways you can work chia seeds into dishes or pair them with foods or drinks:

- **Cereal:** If you pour in milk, almond milk, or so on, it becomes a chia gel, which you don't notice much alongside the cereal.

- **Eggs:** If you're the one cooking them, you can sprinkle the eggs into them; if someone else makes them for you, you can just sprinkle the seeds on top.

- **Danishes or bagels:** The seeds can be sprinkled on top of any butter or cream cheese you put on your danish or bagel. It might be hard to get a whole teaspoonful to stick, but give it a try.

- **Drinks:** A teaspoonful of chia seeds will thicken the drink a bit, but not enough to notice for most drinks. Use trial and error to find out which drinks are the best complement for chia.

- **Sandwiches or burgers:** The seeds can go on top of any condiments you use on sandwiches or burgers. Try for a teaspoonful if you can get it in there.

- **Salads:** These are a great host for chia seeds and aren't that different from other salad toppings.

- **Nuts or chocolate:** You can combine chia seeds with nuts or chocolate to make a trail mix type of snack.

- **Water:** You can put the chia seeds in 10 minutes before, if you like the thicker water. You can also just eat the chia seeds and drink the water separately.

- **Dinner items:** For dinner, you can put chia seeds onto meat, vegetables, or a baked potato or stir it into mashed potatoes or rice.

- **Desserts:** Chia seeds work well as a topping for ice cream, Jell-O, or pudding. You can also easily make a healthy dessert with chia, using its thickening properties to your advantage by mixing the seeds in with almond milk, chocolate milk, and other liquids.

For most of these foods, you're not trying to enhance the flavor—you're just working to get chia seeds in there. Also, you might occasionally end up with a chia seed between your teeth, just as sometimes happens with lettuce or other foods. If you're worried, take a look in the mirror after you eat.

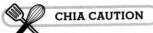 **CHIA CAUTION**

It's embarrassing when a piece of food gets stuck between your teeth—and all too common with chia. Have dental floss handy if you plan to eat chia outside the home.

It takes a little while—and a little bit of water—for chia seeds to form their beneficial gel in your stomach, so get the chia seeds in early in a meal and drink a few ounces of water. Also, remember to eat slowly—a smaller amount of food will make you feel satisfied.

And while you should be aggressive about working dry chia seeds into your own diet, be very cautious about springing it on others you're preparing food for or eating with. Instead of springing it on them unannounced or unasked, let them see you using chia, ask about it, and come to their own conclusions. You don't want to make someone who could become a chia fan into an enemy of chia, especially if he is close to you and affect your own enjoyment of food. Waiting for a request is slower to start with but more likely to create a positive and lasting change for everyone concerned. "Go slow to go fast," as the saying goes.

Making a Gel with Chia

Unlike seeds, chia gel has an additional benefit. You're directly extending your food with a low-calorie, high-fiber, low-cholesterol, nutrient-rich, gluten-free, appetite-suppressing wonder food. This can save you money as well as improving your health.

If you make a gel with chia, you don't have to wait for the dry seeds to combine with water in your stomach when you eat it. The chia gel is already formed and starts moderating your diet right away. So adding a chunk of chia gel to your diet—especially at the start of the day—is a winner both nutritionally and for managing the amount you eat.

You want to make the gel thick. It can be kind of a hassle to add it to foods and eat it, depending on the food. With a thicker gel, you only need a small amount to equal 1 tablespoon of chia seeds.

Here's how to make chia gel:

1. Measure out $^1/_3$ cup, or 5 tablespoons, of chia seeds.

2. Add 2 cups of water to the seeds—if the water is slightly warm, the gel will form more quickly.

3. Put the water plus the seeds into a container with a tight-fitting lid, and shake hard for 15 seconds. Wait a minute, and shake again.

4. Store in the refrigerator. The gel will form in a few hours. The gel will be stable for about two weeks.

It's that easy. Using chia gel is a bit odd until you get used to it. It has almost no flavor, but a consistency like soft Jell-O. As with Jell-O, you'll notice that it's cold.

 SEEDS OF CHANGE

> You don't have to add water as the fluid for your chia gel; you can use fruit or vegetable juices instead. You can also add fruit to your chia gel to make a much healthier version of Jell-O salad or add vegetables to make a kind of cold vegetable soup.

Try to use about ¼ of the chia gel mixture each day in addition to adding dry chia seeds to all sorts of foods. That gets you 1 tablespoon of chia gel from dry seeds and 1 tablespoon from chia gel.

Here are some foods you can put chia gel into and onto fairly unobtrusively:

- Cold cereals or granola
- Hot cereals, such as oatmeal
- Soups
- Drinks
- Salad dressings
- Salsas
- Yogurts
- Cream cheese
- Jams
- Jellies
- Preserves
- Sauces
- Puddings

How much chia gel do you use in these foods? You'll be surprised. Start by adding enough to make the chia gel $^1/_3$ of the total volume—that is, add an amount equal to $^1/_2$ of the food you're adding it to. Eventually, for foods where the chia gel works well for you, you can work your way up to equal amounts of chia gel and the original food.

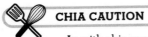 **CHIA CAUTION**

As with chia seeds, if you prepare food for others, don't make others try chia gel unless they want to. Use it in your own food first, even if that means you're heating up your family's tomato soup in two separate saucepans. This lets others "opt in" and make their own choice about adding chia to their own diet.

Using Chia as an Egg Substitute

You can use chia as an egg substitute quite easily:

1. Mix 1 tablespoon of chia with 3 tablespoons of water.

2. Let the chia mixture sit for about 15 minutes.

3. Use the chia mixture in place of one egg.

Chia is more nutritious than most foods, but it isn't more nutritious than eggs. Eggs are a great source of nutrition that's pretty much unmatched as a source of protein, vitamins, and minerals.

Some of the foods for which you can use chia as a partial or complete replacement for eggs include the following:

- Frittatas

- Omelettes

- Meat dishes, such as meatballs

- Cakes

If you—and any people you cook for—eat plenty of meat and other nutrient-dense foods, it won't hurt to drop some of the eggs out of your cooking in favor of chia. But if you are, say, a vegetarian who rations your egg count carefully for the maximum nutritional benefit and protein impact with the minimum harm to other living things, think carefully before taking any eggs out of your diet.

In addition, mouthfeel is a big issue in people's comfort level with food. Eggs serve as a binding agent and thickener for flour and other substances you add them to.

So experiment before using chia to replace eggs in your own food—and experiment twice before using chia to replace eggs in food you fix for others. It might take some trial and error, but over time you might be surprised how many places you can use chia, and the health benefits you get should be rewarding in proportion to your efforts.

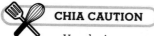 **CHIA CAUTION**

You don't want to create bad associations with chia for yourself or others. Your goal is to incorporate 2 to 3 tablespoons of chia a day in your diet over the long haul. That won't happen if you begin to view chia as a bad thing, or if people you cook and eat with start to see it that way. For example, if you don't like how cupcakes turn out with the chia mixture, it may be better to keep on making your cupcakes with eggs and use the chia mixture in many other places. You don't want to take an aggressive approach early on and not be able to sustain it over time.

Using Chia Flour

Chia flour is simply ground-up chia seeds. Chia seeds are easy to digest without grinding, so there's no nutritional advantage or disadvantage to chia flour. But chia flour is a wonderful alternative to "regular," wheat-based flour for people who want to cut wheat gluten from their diets, add fiber, or just get more nutrition.

You can buy chia flour, or you can make chia flour yourself using a coffee grinder or even a mortar and pestle. It's fun, especially if you have kids who need a project around the house (or if you have kids you want to encourage to play outside by giving them a project to do inside the house).

Here's how you can make it:

1. Pour seeds into a coffee grinder, food processor, or powerful blender.

2. Pulse the seeds until finely ground.

3. Store in an airtight container in a cool, dark spot—or in the refrigerator, if that's the only cool, dark spot you have access to. The flour should last several weeks.

If you look around, you'll see different advice about chia flour. Some say you can just use it as a straight replacement for refined wheat flour, which we believe isn't accurate. Chia flour seems to be more like whole-wheat flour, and as such, it should take about ¾ cup of chia flour to replace 1 cup of refined wheat flour. However, it's a good idea to experiment with the amount of chia flour at least once for yourself and again for anyone you cook for or eat with.

You can try chia flour in any food that requires regular flour, such as the following:

- Breads

- Muffins

- Pancakes

- Tortillas

- Pie crust

- Breadsticks

- Waffles

You can also try it in recipes while using the chia egg substitute, as many flour-based recipes also call for eggs. See what combinations of foods and other chia types work best for you and make you feel like you aren't depriving yourself.

Optimizing Chia Servings

Now that you know how to use chia, how *much* do you use? There are three numbers associated with chia that give us a good idea as to what the maximum and minimum amounts you might want to shoot for: the protein content, the fiber content, and the amount of water chia absorbs.

Chia provides a complete protein, but not in great quantities. One tablespoon of chia seed provides 10 percent of the U.S. Recommended Daily Allowances (RDA) for protein, so you would need to eat 10 tablespoons of chia—or more, if you're pregnant, lactating, or very active—to meet those protein requirements. And if you try to eat 10 tablespoons of chia a day, you run into two other numbers: the fiber content, and the amount of water chia absorbs.

A single tablespoon of chia provides about 40 percent of the fiber you need every day, which is great—especially since most people have diets that are all too poor in fiber. However, if you eat 10 tablespoons of chia, you would get 400 percent of the fiber you need—four times as much. If you're not used to getting even half the fiber you should be getting, suddenly moving even to 100 percent might be a shock to your body. You might become bloated, constipated, or just uncomfortable. And moving to 400 percent might be a much bigger shock.

While fiber isn't toxic, it can be uncomfortable. Therefore, you might want to limit your chia intake initially to 1 tablespoon of chia a day if your weight is closer to 100 pounds, or up to 2 tablespoons a day if your weight is closer to 200 pounds. This way, chia will provide most of your daily fiber needs and a great deal of nutrition as well. When you're comfortable with 1 to 2 tablespoons a day, you can add more chia later.

Water can also affect the way you consume chia. Most people drink too little water and tend to drink it with added substances—caffeine, alcohol, and sugar—that either use up water as the body processes them, take water out of the system by making them want to urinate, or both. Dropping a couple of tablespoons of chia seed into an empty stomach, located in the middle of a water-deprived body, can be uncomfortable. Chia sucks water out of your system, which can leave you feeling bloated, constipated, or just uncomfortable. (And thirsty!) And because chia absorbs nearly 10 times its weight in water, you should be drinking about 8 cups of water a day, or even more.

So taking into account the water and fiber issues, we recommend trying to limit yourself to 2 to 3 tablespoons of chia a day in your diet, with 1 tablespoon's worth of it during breakfast.

 FOOD FOR THOUGHT

> That first tablespoon of chia is special. It not only provides all the nutritional benefits of chia—fiber, antioxidants, omega-3s, minerals, and complete protein, all with little in the way of cholesterol or carbs, and with no gluten—it also forms the famous chia matrix in your stomach.

With chia gel present in your system earlier in the day, everything you eat for breakfast—and for a while afterward—will get absorbed into your body more slowly. You'll feel more energized for longer. You'll also feel less need to rush off to lunch and cram a bunch of bad food into your body to feel full again.

You can increase this effect even more by eating a healthy breakfast, which could be slow-cooked oatmeal, granola, eggs, or chia as an egg substitute. And to top it off, have a few glasses of water in the morning.

The Least You Need to Know

- Beyond foods prepared with chia already in them, you can consume it via chia seeds or chia gel, use it as an egg substitute, and use it in place of flour.
- Adding chia to a food or a meal lowers the effective glycemic index—how fast the body turns food into sugar, which can reduce your chances of developing diabetes.
- One tablespoon of chia seeds gives you 10 percent of your U.S. RDA for protein and 40 percent of your fiber.
- Try to eat 2 to 3 tablespoons of chia a day, with 1 tablespoon of that consumed during breakfast.

Other Chia Products You Can Buy

In the previous chapter, we talked about how getting 2 to 3 tablespoons worth of chia into your diet every day is a worthwhile goal and showed you the main ways to do so— as a seed you add to food, as a gel you add to food, as an egg substitute, and as flour. But that's not all, folks! You can buy premade chia products.

There are two main kinds of chia products. The first kind is other ways to get chia *into* your body, including chia bars, chia-based vitamins, and other foodstuffs. The other type of premade chia products gives you ways to get chia *onto* your body. The rich array of oils in chia, complemented by antioxidants that naturally stabilize them, are a natural (no pun intended) temptation for people making cosmetics, lip balms, toothpaste, and more.

In this chapter, we take you through the different chia products available and their benefits to you.

In This Chapter

- Foods with chia in them
- Chia vitamins
- Chia in cosmetics, creams, and other personal care products

Chia Foods

The following sections discuss different foods that include chia. But first, you should know how much chia is in those products. If you're trying to get 2 tablespoons of chia seeds a day into your diet, as we recommend, then a food with a smattering of chia seeds isn't really going to help you very much.

To figure out how much chia is in a product, check the amount of omega-3 fatty acids in it. Chia is one of the very best sources of omega-3 fatty acids, so marketers will usually put the omega-3 information on the packaging.

One tablespoon of chia has about 2 grams or 2,000 milligrams of omega-3s. So depending on which measurement the company uses on the packaging, you can use "1 tablespoon chia = 2 g or 2,000 mg" as a guideline to calculate the amount of chia included.

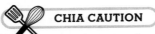

CHIA CAUTION

Product manufacturers smart enough to add chia to their product *might* do a better than average job of adding other good stuff to their products. However, read labels carefully and use online reviews to get the best idea of what's really going on with a product that has chia added to it.

Snack Bars

If you travel or eat out a lot, a snack bar that includes chia is a nice, easy way to bump up your intake. The following are some snack bars that include chia you can look into:

- **Health Warrior Chia Bars** (healthwarrior.com): These bars include 1,000 mg of omega-3s, or about $^1/_2$ tablespoon of chia. They come in a variety of flavors, such as coconut, apple-cinnamon, and even açai berry.

- **muv Bar** (eatuberfoods.com): These bars include about 900 mg of omega-3s, or a little less than $^1/_2$ tablespoon of chia. They come in flavors like cacao, cinnamon, and coconut.

Breakfast Cereals

Breakfast cereals including chia are a good starter product for getting chia into your diet without having to measure out seeds or gel. You can find various kinds of granola, maple clusters, flax and other cereals with chia and other superfoods (such as quinoa) already added. The following are some chia cereals you can check out:

- **Chia-Rezza Organic Chia Cereal** (chia-rezza.com): This cereal includes 3,000 mg of omega-3s, or a hefty $2^1/_2$ tablespoons of chia. It's available in flavors such as almighty mango goji and forbidden fruit.

- **Enjoy Life's Crunchy Flax with Chia** (enjoylifefoods.com/cereals/crunchy-flax-chia/): This cereal includes 1,000 mg of omega-3s, or about $^1/_2$ tablespoon of chia. It's also a great option if you suffer gluten, wheat, dairy, nut, egg, or soy allergies.

- **Kashi Heart to Heart Nutty Chia Flax** (kashi.com/our-foods/cold-cereal/kashi-heart-to-heart-nutty-chia-flax): This cereal includes 320 mg of omega-3s, or about 1 teaspoon of chia. Some reviewers find it a little too sweet, but it's low in sugar and has seven whole grains.

For breakfast cereals in particular, watch out for serving sizes. The amount of omega-3s, calorie counts, and other crucial nutritional information are given per serving size, but the serving sizes used for nutritional information can be quite different from what seems to you like a sensible serving. The best thing to do is to take a measuring cup and measure out what a portion of the cereal looks like according to their guidelines and then measure out what you consider a portion to compare.

Oatmeal

You can find oatmeals that include not only chia but also flax, amaranth, and other good things. The following is an oatmeal that includes chia:

- **Straw Propeller Gourmet Foods' Cherry and Chia Oatmeal** (strawpropellergourmetfoods.com/oatmeal?page=shop.product_details&flypage=flypage. tpl&product_id=22&category_id=1): This oatmeal doesn't have an estimate of its omega-3s. It's on the sugary side, at 18 g, but you could make it an occasional treat.

CHIA CAUTION

Watch out for added sugar and salt in oatmeals. Mainstream foods are packed full of sugar and salt, even some otherwise-healthy products. Sugar can be added "straight" or in the form of maple syrup, honey, and other natural ingredients; regardless, you don't need it. The same goes for salt.

Energy Drinks and Smoothies

You can get nutritional drinks and smoothies with chia added. This is a good thing if you are already drinking this kind of stuff; adding chia to the drinks will slow down the speed with which your body absorbs the sugar in them, which lowers the effective glycemic index. The following are chia energy drink and smoothie options:

- **CHIA/VIE** (drinkchiavie.com): This smoothie includes 2,500 mg of omega-3s, or over 1 tablespoon of chia. This line has a high amount of sugar; it's probably best to try the Mango-J, which has less sugar than the other two in the line.

- **Drink Chia** (drinkchia.com): This energy drink includes 1,100 mg of omega-3s, or a little over $^1/_2$ tablespoon of chia. This brand is passionate about chia, and currently a portion of the proceeds for their lemon-blueberry drink is being donated to a foundation.

If you don't already have drinks of this kind featured in your diet, adding them isn't necessary. Many are likely to contain preservatives and to have lost much of their nutrient value and vitality through the processes of manufacturing, packaging, and shipping. That's not even considering how expensive some of these specialty nutrition drinks can be. As you have for other food options, do your research and check the labels carefully.

Flax and Chia Combinations

Flaxseeds have some of the same advantages of chia seeds and some complementary benefits, such as additional vitamins and minerals. Combining the two together makes for a real nutritional powerhouse. Flax needs to be ground before your body can use it, so unlike with chia seeds, getting a premade product makes sense. If you're considering getting a flax product anyway, getting one that's precombined with chia might make sense. The following are some potential flax and chia products you could try:

- **Carrington Farms' Chia Flax Blend** (carringtonfarms.com/flax-chia-blend-12-oz-pouch/): This blend includes 3,000 mg of omega-3s, or about $1^1/_2$ tablespoons of chia. It can be sprinkled on cereal, yogurt, salad, and other foods.

- **Garden of Life's Organic Golden Flaxseed and Organic Chia Seeds** (gardenoflife.com/Products-for-Life/RAW-Organics/Organic-Golden-Flaxseed-Organic-Chia-Seed.aspx): This blend includes 3,000 mg of omega-3s, or about $1^1/_2$ tablespoons of chia. Like the Carrington Farms blend, this can be sprinkled on foods like cereal, yogurt, and salad.

Whatever you decide on, make sure the product doesn't have whole flaxseeds in it; while whole flaxseeds are nutritious, you don't get the full nutritional benefit unless they're ground.

Chia Vitamins

We recommend that you buy chia in big packages, as described in the next chapter. However, you can also get chia in vitamin-style packaging. This can simply be chia seeds in a small container, usually with a high price per tablespoon, or it can be in the form of capsules with chia oil in them.

I generally don't recommend these kinds of products. They're a lot more expensive than buying chia seed by the pack, and they don't give much advantage. As many of the fish oil tablets on the market, by the time you purchase and use them, the oil may become rancid and/or have spoiled. (This is less of an issue with chia due to the antioxidants it contains, but it's still something to look out for.) Unlike some other beneficial seeds, chia seeds are fully digestible, so the extra processing doesn't really help.

Chia seed oil in softgels might be easier for you to take than actual chia seeds. However, the packaging for the softgels doesn't always list all the nutritional information, so it's hard to tell what's been taken out. Unless you get a prescription or other valued recommendation to take chia seed oil in softgels to fight some specific health problem, you're probably better off simply using the seeds.

There are many different vitamins on the market, so do your research and talk to your doctor about the potential hazards.

 SEEDS OF CHANGE

> If you really like taking softgels, chia oil might be a worthwhile kind to take. Make sure to store them in the refrigerator so the oils in the softgels won't go rancid, and will last longer.

Chia Cosmetics and Creams

Chia oil has its own antioxidants, which helps the chia seed survive and thrive in the desert. Because of these antioxidants, chia oil is very stable and slow to go rancid. This combination of properties makes chia a great base for natural moisturizing creams with no or low levels of artificial ingredients and preservatives and high levels of skin protection.

Chia can be used in exfoliants, moisturizing creams, face washes, and even hair sprays. These products can be made without experimentation on animals or the use of any animal products, making them completely cruelty free. The following are some cosmetics and creams with chia in them.

- **Annamarie Gianni Skincare's Anti-Aging Facial Oil** (shop.annmariegianni.com/Anti-Aging-Facial-Oil-15ml_p_20.html): The combination of chia seed oil and carrot seed oil in this facial oil is said to help rejuvenate the skin.

- **Essensu's Organic Honey Almond Face Scrub** (etsy.com/listing/123919412/organic-raw-honey-almond-gentle-face): The chia seeds in this scrub are said to help exfoliate the skin. It can be used on all skin types.

While chia may be slow to go rancid, that doesn't mean it never does. So once you open a product such as a chia-based skin cream, consider keeping it in a cool, shaded place and using it within a month—or keeping it refrigerated between uses.

Other Personal Care Products with Chia

You can also get chia-infused toothpastes, mouthwashes, and lip balms. Chia can help give texture and body to such products, helping them retain water without being too runny (or hard, in the case of lip balms). You won't get much direct health benefit from any chia you might accidentally ingest with these products, but you also won't be exposed to animal products or chemicals that might have been used to make other versions of these items instead. Here are some other products you can find that include chia:

- **Chia Serum** (perriconemd.com/product/chia+serum.do): This serum combines chia oil and vitamins. Add it to shampoo, skin cream, and other products to bring the smoothness and richness of chia into the mix.

- **Mama Bear Skin Care Peppermint Stick Lip Balms** (mamabearskincare.com/lip-balms.html): This lip balm is said to be cooling and refreshing, with peppermint and spearmint oils as well as chia.

- **Vitacare Sensitive Whitening Toothpaste** (amazon.com/Sensitive-Whitening-Toothpaste-Mint-Extract/dp/B008R2UM92): This toothpaste includes a chia mint extract. It is said to help relieve tooth sensitivity and moisturize dry mouths.

 SEEDS OF CHANGE

When shopping for chia-based products, we recommend starting with online sources for trying a range of chia products, unless you happen to spot something attractive locally. Online shopping gives you a wide range of choices, online reviews, and lower prices. Once you identify—and perhaps try—products you like, consider buying them from retailers who are in line with your values. This can be an online shopping site that promotes natural and organic products or a local retailer that's willing to listen to your personal requests.

The Least You Need to Know

- Chia comes in snack bars, breakfast cereals, smoothies, vitamins, face creams, and more.
- You can get chia in vitamin form, though it can sometimes be too overly processed by manufacturers.
- Chia has valuable oils that are good building blocks for all kinds of products—and even more valuable natural antioxidants that stabilize the oils without artificial chemicals.

Stocking Up for the Chia Seed Diet

Chia is a superfood, with so many good qualities—and so few bad ones—that people can hardly have too much of it in their diet.

Chia is particularly suited to modern culture, as people tend to have way too much calorie-rich food available and way too little fiber. Chia is low in calories, moderates your desire for food of all types, and provides ample amounts of fiber. In combination with other healthy foods, you can be on your way to a fitter and healthier you.

In this chapter, we discuss the ideal foods and drinks for the chia seed diet and provide a shopping list to set you on the right path.

In This Chapter

- What sort of foods you should eat
- Don't forget drinks!
- A shopping plan for your diet

Eating Food on the Chia Seed Diet

Michael Pollan, author of *The Omnivore's Dilemma,* sums up his credo in just four words: "Eat food. Mostly plants." What does he mean by this?

The term *food* when referring to people's diets is broad beyond belief. Humans are the ultimate omnivores. Omnivores have a mix of herbivore and carnivore features—and the mix can tell us what a given creature has evolved to eat. People's teeth are a mix of herbivore (molar) and carnivore (incisor) teeth. So humans plainly evolved to eat a wide mix of foods; lots of plants and, relatively speaking (compared to other omnivores, including other primates), lots of meat.

FOOD FOR THOUGHT

Your best and easiest technique for adopting chia into your diet depends significantly on the diet you're starting with. Try to make the least change that you need to in order to accomplish your goals. For example, if bread is something that's not a huge staple in your diet, make it a goal to watch your consumption of it. At a restaurant, you can avoid the bread basket or simply have one slice. When you have a sandwich, you can take a slice of bread off the top of each half and then glom the bottoms together to make a thicker sandwich that has a greater proportion of the "stuff" in the middle and a much lower proportion of bread.

For example, Eskimos live much of their lives from eating only the meat and other body parts of seals. Europeans have adapted genetically to drink milk that is developed in cows' bodies to feed their own offspring. Then there are people who subsist largely on insects, at least part of the year, while others avoid eating them as much as possible. Some people are entirely vegetarian—of necessity (due to the food that's available to them), for religious reasons, or by choice.

The second part of Pollan's dictum, "mostly plants," limits his suggestion as to what you should eat the most of by quantity, while not excluding any specific food at all. This relates to the chia seed diet, in that you should really consume as much beyond the processed foods readily available as possible—but not try to eliminate foods entirely.

Instead, you can use an approach to eating well called *crowding out.* You add lots of the foods you want to be eating to your diet, basing your meals and recipes on these desirable foods. This gradually reduces, and then even eliminates, less-healthy foods from your diet while still letting you consume what you need to feel full.

Cruise your local farmers' market, organic market, or supermarket looking for in-season, fresh vegetables to add to your shopping basket. You can then use this book, other cookbooks, friends and family, and the Internet to find recipes that help you use the foods you find.

Following are a few examples of healthy foods you will run into and how you can use them to "crowd out" less-healthy foods from your diet:

- **Salad mix:** Many local farmers' markets feature salad mixes that include several different kinds of greens and—I kid you not—flowers, all premixed. Buying this mix makes it very easy for you to have at least one salad a day while cutting your prep time in half. If you enjoy making your own salads from scratch and have the time to do it, great. Otherwise, buy salad mix and use it at least once a day.

- **Spaghetti squash:** This is a hearty squash that you bake. The insides then come out in a stringy form that's easy to eat and serves as a replacement for pasta. Spaghetti squash plus spaghetti sauce makes for a healthy main course for any meal.

- **Big and small squashes:** There's a wide variety of squashes of all sizes, shapes, and colors. You can slice them and add them to salads or steam them and use them for a hearty main dish. Every different breed and color has its own nutritional profile.

- **Eggplant:** Eggplant is so rich in flavor, with a meaty, tangy taste, that you can use it as a main course in a meatless—or less-meat—meal. Eggplant can be runny, so work to find and use recipes that have a texture you like.

- **Organic, free-range eggs:** The right kind of eggs have much more nutrition than factory-farmed eggs that only match the good ones in fat and cholesterol. Try making omelettes with one egg per person, using chia and water to stretch the single egg into a hearty frittata or omelette.

- **Organically raised meat:** As with "good eggs," organically raised meat goes twice as far per ounce as the mainstream stuff. Buy small, high-quality steaks and ground lamb or pork instead of hamburger. Use half as much (which makes the price per serving about the same) and enjoy it twice as much.

- **Wild-caught fish:** Farmed fish tend to live in water that has more fish waste in it, and the farmed fish aren't as likely to swim much, so their muscle tone is poor. Wild-caught fish come from clean water and have stronger muscles, and therefore more nutrition and less fat.

 SEEDS OF CHANGE

A big strategy for eating better is to eat much better food in somewhat smaller quantities. Chia is a huge help in this strategy as it stretches dishes, adds nutrition, and fills your stomach.

Chia and What You Drink

We've talked a lot in this book about drinking water, especially as a complement anytime you eat chia seeds. We also have several recipes for chia drinks in this book (see Chapter 15). But what about all the other things you drink?

Modern drinking habits are your enemy when it comes to getting and staying healthy. The "supersize me" approach doesn't just apply to soft drinks. People used to treat fruit juices as a superfood, drinking tiny glasses of freshly squeezed juice. Now they drink huge glasses of processed, refrigerated juice with preservatives. People also drink huge coffees with milk and other ingredients that run the calorie count into the stratosphere.

As you get started, try adding a teaspoon of chia to all your drinks. Some of them will work well for you, while others won't. The experimentation will be fun and will teach you a lot of ways to add chia to your diet.

Also, consider moderating your intake of alcohol. It's easy to gain a pound or two a year from less than 100 extra calories a day. That's about the number of calories in one beer or one glass of wine. (They don't call extra weight in the stomach area a "beer belly" for nothing!) Alcoholic drinks are full of empty calories, which makes it nearly impossible to lose weight when consumed regularly.

If you exercise regularly (see Chapter 9), you have a fighting chance and somewhat more room in your diet for a drink here or there. But for the start of the chia seed diet, you need to avoid canceling it out with an extra drink or two here and there. When you reach your target weight or have started getting the benefits you want, you can then start adding the occasional drink back in.

Keep your drink sizes small for every drink except water. Adding chia will make you thirsty—fill that need with water.

Stocking Other Items for the Chia Seed Diet

To make planning and preparing healthy meals a bit easier beyond adding chia, it's a good idea to have a decent collection of basic ingredients on hand so that, come shopping time, all you need to worry about are the base ingredients recipes call for—the meats, veggies, and so on.

The following is a list of staple items beyond chia you should have on hand. It's certainly not all-inclusive, but it should give you a good start on healthier eating. And of course, if we've included ingredients you just don't like, you don't have to stock them.

SEEDS OF CHANGE

Having your pantry and fridge stocked with healthy staples gives you a jump-start on meal planning and helps you resist binging due to not having the right foods in the house.

For your pantry:

Breads, grains, pastas:

- ❏ Whole-wheat tortillas
- ❏ Whole-grain pasta in different shapes and sizes
- ❏ Oats, old-fashioned or quick-cooking
- ❏ Plain instant oatmeal packets
- ❏ Long-grain rice
- ❏ Brown rice
- ❏ Whole-grain bread
- ❏ Whole-grain crackers, regular or low-sodium
- ❏ Unseasoned breadcrumbs
- ❏ Couscous
- ❏ Quinoa

Spices and seasonings:

- ❏ Cinnamon
- ❏ Nutmeg
- ❏ Ground ginger
- ❏ Black pepper
- ❏ Onion powder
- ❏ Garlic powder
- ❏ Minced onion
- ❏ Table salt
- ❏ Sea salt
- ❏ Crushed red pepper flakes
- ❏ Paprika
- ❏ Garlic chile sauce or hot sauce
- ❏ Mustard

Baking:

- ❏ Brown sugar
- ❏ Granulated sugar
- ❏ Honey
- ❏ Vanilla extract
- ❏ Peanut butter
- ❏ Agar powder
- ❏ Flavored gelatin mixes
- ❏ All-purpose flour
- ❏ Whole-wheat flour
- ❏ Splenda

Oils and dressings:

- ❏ Canola oil
- ❏ Extra-virgin olive oil
- ❏ Reduced-sodium soy sauce
- ❏ Nonstick cooking spray

Vegetables:

- ❏ Onions
- ❏ Bell peppers (red and green)
- ❏ Carrots
- ❏ Bibb lettuce
- ❏ Spaghetti squash
- ❏ Potatoes

Canned goods:

- ❏ Canned tomatoes
- ❏ Canned beans, preferably low sodium
- ❏ Canned tuna, packed in water
- ❏ Canned (or boxed) low-sodium chicken, beef, vegetable stock or broth

Dried fruits and nuts:

- ❏ Dried raisins, cranberries, cherries, and other fruits
- ❏ Various types of nuts

For your refrigerator:

- ❏ Skim or 1 percent milk
- ❏ Soy milk
- ❏ Almond milk
- ❏ Plain fat-free Greek yogurt
- ❏ Reduced-fat cheddar cheese
- ❏ Vegan margarine spread
- ❏ Reduced-fat sour cream
- ❏ Reduced-fat cream cheese
- ❏ Reduced-fat salad dressing
- ❏ Reduced-fat mayonnaise
- ❏ Large eggs

For your freezer:

- ❏ Vegetables with no added sauces
- ❏ Fruit with no added sugar

The Least You Need to Know

- Aim for 2 to 3 tablespoons of chia seeds in your diet each day, depending on your weight.
- The chia seed diet is not about eliminating foods, but changing your habits so your diet is made up more of healthy options.
- Use the shopping list to help you have the ingredients and foods on hand to be successful on the diet.

Preparing for the Chia Seed Diet

What you eat is a huge part of your lifestyle. Diet affects—and is affected by—all your relationships, your work, your exercise patterns (or non-exercise patterns), how well or poorly you sleep, and much more.

This part shows how chia seeds can help you find a healthy balance in your diet, eating only the calories you need while packing in high levels of nutrition into almost every bite of food and sip of liquids you take.

Chia is relatively unobtrusive, but any change you make in your diet can feel like a hassle—and even more so if it changes how you eat with others. And if you prepare food for other people, or eat food they prepare, you need to figure out how much to go along with them and how much to ask them to go along with you. Therefore, this part also helps you with challenges related to eating outside the home during a typical day, to travel, and to eating with others.

Finally, this part introduces the chia meal two-week diet for both 1,500- and 2,000-calorie diets. This is a core asset of the book; if you use it wisely, it can help change your life. The two-week diet contains everything you need to lose weight, to maintain a healthy weight, and to develop new habits that you can benefit from for the rest of your life.

Lifestyle Changes and Weight Management

Your goal in taking on a chia-based diet is probably not to demonstrate your love for the chia plant or its seeds, nor is it just to do something that sounds catchy or looks interesting. You're probably looking to lose weight (or maintain a healthy weight, if you're already there) and to have better overall health.

One key reason chia can serve as the basis of an entire diet much more than other foods—even other superfoods—is because of its ability to form a matrix in your stomach that slows the absorption of all the food you eat. So it's not about displacing most other foods; it's about reducing the total amount of food you feel you need to eat, while providing you a comfortable feeling of fullness and steady energy throughout the day.

There's also another side to losing weight and maintaining good health, which is exercise. To a greater degree than most foods, chia is relevant for exercise.

In this chapter, we'll briefly describe the modern problems you encounter with modern foods and processing and how they can affect your health. We then show you how chia, in conjunction with exercise, can set you on a path to better health.

In This Chapter

- Health problems you may encounter with certain foods
- How processed foods can further diminish nutritional value and affect your diet
- Chia as an aid to weight loss
- Boosting your energy for exercise with chia

The Negative Consequences of Certain Foods on the Modern Diet

People's desires for food evolved at a time when food was scarce, and sweet and salty foods indicated nutritional deficits that almost everyone had. Sweet foods, such as honey and ripe fruits, were rich sources of calories and other nutritional goodness. Salt features an element—sodium— you need in your daily diet.

However, the very high availability and very low cost of mass-produced food have made people less healthy, whether through overconsumption or allergies.

Milk and Dairy

Milk and dairy products are rich in nutrients, but also rich in calories and fats, which can lead to weight gain. For example, cheese is very high in calories and fat. A lot of popular cheeses today— such as American cheese—also have very little flavor, so it's easy to pile on the cheese.

Most grown people in the world also can't easily digest milk or dairy products, because they lack an enzyme that breaks down lactose, the key sugar in milk.

 FOOD FOR THOUGHT

You can purchase products such as Lactaid to break down lactose for you,. You just have to be conscientious about eating them in the same meal as milk, cheese, and so on.

Wheat and Rice

Wheat-based products—and, to a lesser extent, foods containing rice—are also problematic. Wheat and rice were cultivated widely only in the last few thousand years, and over time entire nations have become largely dependent on these two grains as foods. They both contain gluten, which many people have an allergy to called *celiac disease.*

In addition to celiac disease, many people are more or less intolerant of gluten, especially wheat gluten. As with dairy products, wheat gluten is found in many products where one wouldn't expect it, because the gluten in wheat is useful for helping prepared foods stick together. For instance, pizza is full of gluten, causing a lot of regret for people on gluten-free diets. Even many salad dressings have gluten.

Refined Sugar

Sugar isn't new overall, but refined sugar is. Widespread refining and trading of sugar has only become common in the last few centuries. It's useful as a preservative, but it also adds a seemingly desirable flavor not only to traditionally sugary foods, such as cakes, but also to other unexpected products, such as ketchups.

Refined sugar gives people a little buzz when they eat it, which can lead to eating more foods with sugar in higher quantities to continue getting that happy buzz. Also, because refined sugar is so pure, it's composed entirely of empty calories; therefore, the processed and prepared foods that get most of their calories from sugar are largely made up of empty calories as well, meaning they don't provide much value to people's diets.

Salt

As with sugar, salt is an excellent preservative. It also adds what people think of as a desirable flavor to almost any food. Ketchup is just one food that's pumped full of salt, and many foods have both salt and sugar in abundance.

Salt is full of sodium, which causes inflammation in the body's tissues, notably the coronary arteries. Inflamed arteries build up plaque, restricting blood flow. The result: high blood pressure, which is unhealthy in many ways, including that it increases people's risk of a heart attack.

Salt also has an odd property that's different from many other foods—people develop a tolerance for the taste, meaning they need more and more salt to feel a "salty" taste in food. Once people develop a high salt tolerance, they're insensitive to the large amounts of salt in processed food, restaurant meals, and so on, leading to getting too much sodium in the diet.

 FOOD FOR THOUGHT

Salt has been used for a long time as a natural preservative, so people's affinity for salt might have developed as a way to help them stay away from rotten meat.

How Modern Processing and Farming Practices Can Make Foods Worse for You

As you read in the previous section, certain foods alone can cause health problems when consumed too much, but processing can make them even worse for your diet.

Processed foods have been developed for things that people think of as positive: purity (such as white sugar and white flour), long shelf life, and ease of use in cooking. They also appeal disproportionately to people's desire for sweet and salty foods.

There's even a more subtle addictive factor to processed foods. Complex starches, such as those in yams, take time for the body to break down into sugars (which is what the body really wants). But simple starches, such as those in a "pure" white potato, break down very quickly in the body, yielding their sugars very rapidly. These simple starches, which are in a lot of processed foods, make those foods gain an addictive quality. For example, when you eat white bread, you quickly get a little rush of energy; once that energy is gone, you need to eat again quickly. The body wants that little rush of (internally developed) sugar again and again; eating then becomes not just about the stomach being empty, but also wanting to consume more of that food again. This rush from simple starchy foods is the same as what happens with sugar, but people don't recognize it as such because the starch doesn't taste sweet when they eat it.

Processed foods are also full of preservatives and chemically produced "nutrients" that look good on a box label but don't represent the overall nutritional value that the same nutrients represent when found in nonprocessed foods. And that brings us to a major problem with nonprocessed foods: Many don't have the same nutritional value as they used to. Modern apples, for instance, are bred for toughness in shipping, not maximum nutrition, and are grown in poor soils depleted by modern farming practices.

So, many processed foods are almost devoid of nutrition, meaning nonprocessed foods have to carry nearly all the burden of getting nutrients and fiber into people's diets—but nonprocessed foods aren't what they used to be.

Eating nonprocessed foods in a higher proportion than processed foods is obviously the answer, but it can be tough. In most cultures, processed food sets the tone for how people eat. Going out a great deal, eating on the go, very fast food preparation times—these are all expectations of a processed-food culture that are hard to match with nonprocessed foods. But while the processed foods may be cheaper and easier to get in the short run, the health problems caused by an unhealthy diet—such as weight gain, reduced energy, and allergy issues—are very expensive indeed.

 FOOD FOR THOUGHT

I strongly recommend Michael Pollan's best-known book, *The Omnivore's Dilemma,* which describes how a creature with our evolutionary roots can be best served by choosing carefully from the foods available to people today. He also describes the immense role of corn and, to a lesser extent, soybeans within the ingredients list of most processed food. Pollan's book is likely to help you a great deal in moving to a healthier diet.

Moving Away from Sedentary Practices

Cross-cultural studies of different groups, living at different levels of technology, have shown it's very common for people of all cultures to spend at least two hours a day moving—whether going to and from work, visiting, getting food and water, or for other reasons. In most cultures, most of that movement time is spent walking.

However, motorized transportation, particularly cars, cuts into that. Your movement time becomes sitting time. The changing nature of work and housework has also contributed to a more sedentary lifestyle. Labor-saving machinery saves chances to burn calories, and staring at a computer screen is not only not very active, it can also cause health problems, such as repetitive stress injuries and back problems. Studies have shown that sitting for any length of time each day, whether in a car or at your desk, is actually bad for your health and longevity.

And when you add food to the mix, it has an even bigger impact. People are built to take in about 4,000 or 5,000 calories a day and then use just half of it running their basic bodily machinery. Active people who use 4,000 to 5,000 calories a day can afford a lot of mistakes. Their diet can have a lot of relatively empty calories in it, as long as half or so of it is nutritious, because they'll still get the nutrients they need out of the nutritious half.

But if you're one of the many who's sedentary, you only have a budget of 2,000 to 2,500 calories if you're not to overeat. Because of this, you can't afford to blow any of that on unhealthy food. It's difficult to avoid, because unhealthy food is prominent, really convenient, and marketed constantly. In fact, many Americans eat one fast food meal every day and eat most of those meals in their—wait for it—cars.

When you're sedentary, your body loses muscle mass, which in turn makes your actual calorie requirements and ability to exercise decline over time. As your calorie budget for getting the nutrients you need becomes less and less, you're likely to become undernourished, underexercised, and unhealthy, in a declining spiral.

You need to either become a sedentary paragon of virtue, eating only what's perfect—which is pretty hard to do—or step up your game and get active. It only takes about an hour a day of movement to make a big difference in your calorie balance, giving you a little room to work with for losing weight or eating some suboptimal food at times.

Changing Your Dietary Habits and Losing Weight with Chia

So how can chia help? Chia is great for losing weight—or maintaining an already healthy weight—because it forms a gel in your stomach, taking up room and moderating the pace at which your body digests food. Chia is also a steady source of energy. As the gel slowly breaks down, your body gets a steady flow of food.

Aztec warriors and Native American runners and traders used chia to help them keep going on long marches, on long runs, and in battle. A small pouch of chia seeds, taken with plenty of water, could keep them going for a day or more. But this doesn't just apply to active individuals. You can use chia to both give you that kind of sustainable energy and also slow the absorption of other food, making what you eat into a longer-term fuel source.

If you're just starting to move away from a sedentary lifestyle and are trying to steer clear or limit processed foods, you'll find chia will help you stay energized and feel fuller longer. Let's take a deeper look at how chia can help you lose weight and improve your health—and what you can do to help it along.

How Chia Can Help You

If you eat chia in the amount of 1 to 2 tablespoons a day, you can get much of the benefit of lap band surgery—without the band or the surgery!

The gel that forms in your stomach from chia does three awesome things that are beneficial for weight loss and your health:

1. It takes up a lot of space in your stomach, making the effective capacity of your stomach less. This, in turn, makes you not want to eat as much.

2. It slows the absorption of the food you do eat. The food then takes longer to digest, making you feel fuller longer.

3. It provides lots of fiber— more than half your daily needs, if you eat roughly 1 tablespoon of chia for every 100 pounds you weigh. Most people today eat too little fiber, which is bad for the digestive tract, for potentially developing diabetes, and more. Chia provides that missing fiber, which helps soaks up toxins and takes them out of your body while giving your insides much-needed exercise.

A final, smaller benefit of chia is that it makes you take in more water, whether as part of chia gel, drinking it while eating chia seeds (to prevent feeling thirsty), or drinking it after eating chia seeds (because you feel thirsty). Additional water, like additional fiber, is great for your system— washing out toxins and helping every cell in your body work better while filling you up and reducing hunger.

 CHIA CAUTION

It takes some time to adjust to regular use of chia, so watch your intake of food. When you first start, you may tend to eat the same amount of food as you were used to eating. This can make you overeat and then feel bloated or overly full. Over time, you'll learn how to cut down your meal sizes to feel sated but not too full.

What You Can Do to Make Chia More Effective

Chia is a diet booster. If you're carrying extra weight and add chia to your diet, you might stop gaining weight—or even start slowly losing. If you do go on a diet—or even better, a diet and exercise plan (see the next section in this chapter)—chia will help you keep your portions moderate and help you feel good during and after exercising.

Sadly, however, chia isn't a miracle weight-loss food; you'll need to make some minor adjustments to make sure you're getting all of those nutritional and weight-loss benefits. Here are a few simple steps you can make it more effective:

1. **Use chia frequently.** Make sure you constantly put chia into different foods and drinks. Not only will that allow you to experiment with textures related to adding chia, you'll also get more chances to feel its benefits.

2. **Use chia consistently.** Your body will help you here; once you're using chia a lot, you'll feel it when you don't. Plan to have chia with just about every meal, especially breakfast and lunch—that way, you'll be set up for the day.

3. **Learn to listen to your body.** The Western way of eating teaches people to cram tons of food into their mouths the moment they feel hungry. Chia can help you avoid that urge, but you have to enforce it. You may sometimes feel like stopping by your favorite fast-food restaurant, but the way you'll probably feel after eating it won't be as satisfying as before the chia seed diet.

4. **Eat most of your food—and then take a break.** Your body delays letting you know you're full until 15 or 20 minutes after you've in fact consumed enough to feel satisfied. This little trick your body plays to encourage you to overeat when food is available so you're ready for droughts, famines, and so on is more likely today to make you gradually get heavier instead. By taking a break from your meals, you give your feeling of fullness a chance to catch up.

5. **Drink plenty of water.** Most people don't drink enough water anyway, mistaking it for hunger and eating instead of drinking. Chia works much better for you when you drink extra water just to hydrate it, but doing this will also keep you hydrated, too.

Chia and Exercise

As you learned earlier in this chapter, chia is a way to boost your energy and get you up and moving. It should be no surprise, then, that chia works very well with any exercise program.

Exercise used to be part of daily life. Walking was the only way to get anywhere; running could get you there faster. Horses were an alternative for some, but even horseback riding involves a fair amount of exertion. Most jobs or chores involved a fair amount of effort as well. Just the movement involved in washing dishes, sweeping, or beating carpets added to people's strength and their use of the calories in their food.

Now, exercise is seen as a hassle. The extra clothes and cleaning up involved, plus the packed nature of most people's days, make it a task that's very easy indeed to put off. However, by getting active and incorporating chia into your exercise program, you can improve your health and lose or maintain a healthy weight.

Whether you're already active or just getting started, the following discusses some popular forms of exercise and how you can use chia with them to get the greatest benefit.

 SEEDS OF CHANGE

One of the biggest problems people can have when combining a diet with a new exercise regimen is that their body wants to eat more than enough to make up for the exercise benefit, which can lead to overeating. Chia keeps releasing energy into your body steadily over a long period of time, giving you that extra surge of energy and helping to control your appetite.

Walking

Walking is a pretty easy exercise habit to get into. In terms of footfalls, at least one foot is always on the ground. It takes about 20 minutes to cover 1 mile while walking, so you're going 3 miles an hour. Because you're moving slowly, your brain can handle navigational challenges while walking without you consciously giving them much thought.

We personally believe you should walk at least one hour a day. Designing your life so you walk this much without any extra effort is a major accomplishment. One favored way to do it is to get walking in the morning, so you don't have a chance to defer it later in the day.

Chia is a great energy boost for walking. You don't need to do anything special—just get in your 1 to 2 tablespoons a day of chia, hopefully most of it in your breakfast and lunch. You can even go walking immediately after eating without much risk of upsetting yourself. The steady energy provided by chia will help you regardless of when you decide to get in your walking.

Jogging

Jogging is a very slow run. When jogging, you have both feet off the ground a small—possibly very small—part of the time. (There is a sort of "jog-shuffle" that keeps one foot on the ground all of the time, but this is preparation for jogging, rather than the true thing itself.) When jogging, you move about twice as fast as walking, covering 1 mile in 10 to 12 minutes, or 5 to 7 miles an hour.

If you're not an experienced jogger, make sure you follow these guidelines to jog safely and effectively:

- Wear shoes with great support. You want to make your feet as comfortable as possible to reduce soreness and potential injury.

- Stretch so your muscles are loose and warm. This can help you avoid any pulled muscles.

- Warm up a bit by doing some walking first. Also, consider walking one minute out of every seven or eight minutes, to give yourself a breather and change it up a bit.

FOOD FOR THOUGHT

A famous definition of jogging is that it's running slowly enough that you can still hold a conversation. If you're out of shape, you won't be able to do that—and that's okay. Do what you can; you'll benefit, and over time, you'll get faster.)

Unlike with walking, it's good to be a bit more thoughtful about your chia and other food consumption before jogging. Consider having a snack with chia in it about one hour before you start your jog, as the more-strenuous exercise could make you feel sick to your stomach. Also, drink lots of water in the two hours or so before jogging, but don't tank up on water just before starting. Like the food, anything you chug down just before jogging might come back up if you go long or hard in your workout.

By supplementing your jogging program with chia, your stomach will neither be cavernously empty nor dangerously full while exercising. The food you ate and the chia in your stomach will provide you with steady energy while you're jogging and keep you from getting ravenously hungry during or just after your jog.

Running

Running is a high-impact exercise, as small areas on your feet are striking the ground and carrying the full weight of your body. You're also moving at a fast-enough speed that you can't comfortably talk. When you run, you can cover 1 mile in about 7 minutes and 8 to 15 miles in an hour. Because it's so high impact, many people avoid running; however, many others swear by it (when they're not swearing at it).

When running, it's important to paying attention to details to reduce injuries and maximize the benefits. As with walking and jogging, you need shoes with good support. You also need to choose your running surfaces carefully—avoid concrete entirely, minimize running on asphalt, and try for dirt or grass. The latter are softer surfaces that are less likely to lead to injury.

Good nutrition is also key to running, and here chia is a huge help. Many runners "carbohydrate load" in the hours before a big run or a race so they have plenty of calories to draw on while running. Chia provides energy of its own and draws out the body's absorption of other food while running. In fact, vegetarian and vegan runners—who have to pay extra attention to diet, nutrition, and energy usage—are often among the biggest athletic proponents of chia. Just make sure to consume it an hour or so before running to avoid nausea during your run.

Swimming

Swimming is in many ways the best exercise. It's quite safe (assuming you know how to swim!) and very low impact. You can do it for a long time, burning tons of calories and building your muscles, with little risk of injury.

Swimming burns calories partly because water is much more efficient than air at wicking heat away from your body. That's because water is much denser than air, so more cool-water molecules strike your body, take a little heat away, and then bounce off. This cumulative effect multiplies the calorie-burning impact of swimming. But it can also chill you and make you end your workout before you'd like it to be over.

This is where chia is perfect. By slowly releasing its own energy and other food energy, chia can help you swim longer, faster, and without discomfort, simply because your muscles don't get as tired.

Try consuming chia at least an hour before your swimming workout (to avoid any cramps or discomfort brought on by the exercise), and see if you can feel the difference.

SEEDS OF CHANGE

Drink plenty of water before swimming; you should also drink water during your swim if you go for more than about 20 minutes. Running out of water doesn't always register as thirst, especially when you're surrounded by water, but it can make you tired and despondent without necessarily knowing why.

Bike Riding

Bike riding is excellent low-impact exercise—as long as you avoid crashing, of course. Chia can help you keep going faster and longer.

Bike riding is usually an endurance sport, and the longer you can keep going, the more benefit you'll get. Chia helps keep the fires burning so you enjoy a bike ride for longer.

As with other sports, give yourself an hour between eating and the start of a ride. You'll appreciate the long-lasting impact of chia when others are lagging behind.

Martial Arts

Chia was famously used by Aztec warriors to stay strong in battle. It's great for supporting the intensity and focus needed to perform well—and to stay healthy—in martial arts workouts, sparring, and competition.

If you're a dedicated martial artist, you're probably quite aware of your body. Consider trying chia in different forms and quantities to see what feels best and best supports different workouts, sparring sessions, and competitive sessions.

Chia seems particularly appropriate for competitions with multiple sessions or uncertain start times. Steady, long-lasting energy is a priority here, and chia is just what a martial artist needs to help fill in any gaps in sustenance.

SEEDS OF CHANGE

If you're just starting out in an aerobics or other exercise class, one of the toughest things can be finding yourself struggling to keep up with the already super-fit people. Instead of getting discouraged, make sure you consume some chia about an hour before class; the steady flow of energy you get from it will help you when you're mixing up various intense moves and varying numbers of repetitions.

And don't forget to drink lots of water—if an aerobics class or other workout class doesn't make you sweat, you're probably not doing it right!

The Least You Need to Know

- Chia can help you reduce or eliminate potentially troublesome foods, food components, and spices such as dairy, meat, wheat gluten, salt, and sugar.
- Chia is a great source of fiber and can help you feel fuller longer, making it a nice weight-loss booster.
- Consuming chia before you exercise can give you an extra burst of energy to accomplish your workout.

CHAPTER 10

Beating Chia Seed Diet Challenges

Staying on any diet is tough, and the chia seed diet is no exception. Between busy schedules, lack of energy, and other daily obstacles, it can be difficult to keep up the enthusiasm and motivation for a diet over a long period of time. But we're here to help.

In this chapter, we give you ways to deal with the potential challenges you could face on the chia seed diet.

In This Chapter

- Making chia part of a busy schedule
- Focusing on your body and the food you consume
- Curbing the secondary effects of chia

Chia on the Go

Like any diet, it's easier to follow the chia diet when you're at home and have time on your hands. However, in this fast-paced world, it's not always that simple. Between working, doing errands, and taking the kids to school, it can be easy to just grab fast food for a meal.

However, there are quick and easy ways to get chia seeds into your diet every day and keep on a healthy path. The following are some suggestions for getting chia into your meals and resisting temptation when you're away from home.

Starting Your Day Off Right

To be successful on the chia seed diet, you need to do some planning. First thing in the morning is a good time to think about what you'd like to eat during the day or even during the week (see Chapter 11 for some sample two-week meal plans). It's also a good idea to figure out some snacks you can have on hand to "tough it out" if you have to go an extra hour or two between healthy meals, as those are the times when it can be easy to cheat. By thinking about what challenges you could potentially face, you can be more proactive in your diet.

The morning also includes a very important meal for the chia seed diet: breakfast. The key to having a good day on your diet is eating a solid, on-plan breakfast including chia. Here are some quick and easy options for breakfast (see Chapter 14 for breakfast recipes):

- Have a bowl of granola with ¼ cup of chia gel in it. That's enough to provide you with a tablespoon worth of chia seeds to start the day.

- Fix an omelette with two eggs and 1 tablespoon of chia seeds, and put a few ounces of extra milk in the egg and chia mix to provide liquid for the chia seeds to soak up. This tastes really good and hearty; the chia seeds don't add a strong flavor, but what they do provide actually seems to improve the taste of the omelette.

- Fix an omelette with one egg, 1 tablespoon of chia seeds, and 3 tablespoons of water. This makes one egg do the work of two and also provides the base for a pretty good omelette.

- If you need to pick up something outside of home for breakfast, pick a healthy option, and mix in some chia seeds. McDonald's oatmeal is one breakfast food you can mix chia with and have a filling, healthy breakfast (see Chapter 12).

Having the needed foods for these alternatives handy can be a fair amount of work but really rewarding. Especially on days you get up a bit late, having a plan for breakfast and other meals will make it easier to start your day off right. Add in an hour or so of exercise, and you've gotten ahead on your goals for the day by a good amount.

If you rush out of the house without breakfast—and without time to plan your other meals—it's hard to have a good day, diet-wise.

FOOD FOR THOUGHT

A popular recent book is called *VB6*, short for "Vegan Before 6". The author, Mark Bittman, is a food writer for the *New York Times*. He suggests being vegan before 6 P.M. and doing whatever you want for dinner, dessert, and any late-night events. Bittman lost 15 pounds in a month on this approach, which has to be unusual, but you might have at least some success on a chia-infused version of the VB6 approach. So try using the *VB6* approach with the suggestions and recipes in this book.

Having Snacks and Chia with You During the Day

Chia is wonderful while it lasts. Any meal with chia will fill you up faster than you might expect and keep you feeling full for several hours. However, even the gel that chia forms gets broken down at some point—usually a few hours after your last meal. At this point, you may experience a sudden rush of hunger. If you're not at home or busy rushing around, how do you curb your cravings?

To control your hunger without overindulging, carry healthy snacks you can nibble on throughout the day. An ideal snack is a mix of unsalted, uncooked nuts and well-made dark chocolate. For example, a snack of about 15 uncooked, unsalted almonds is boring enough to help keep you from eating more, but tasty and filling enough to be satisfying. And when it comes to the dark chocolate, you don't have to break the bank—you can make eight squares last four days by having a single snack of two squares of chocolate each day. Eaten this way, the fancy chocolate is less expensive than filling the gap in your eating schedule with a less-expensive—and less healthy—milk-chocolate candy bar.

SEEDS OF CHANGE

If you're not too far—in space or in time—from refrigeration, you can have a snack of Greek yogurt with 1 teaspoon of chia seeds. Another option is a smoothie with 1 teaspoon of chia seeds which works in the same way; the chia seeds ameliorate any blood sugar surge you might otherwise get from the smoothie. However, these particular snacks, which include dairy—and, for the smoothie option, fruit—are less likely to fit some diets than almonds or dark chocolate.

And make sure you always carry chia with you. You can place 1 or 2 tablespoons of chia seeds in a plastic zipper-lock bag or other container to carry with you, depending on space. I suggest 1 or 2 tablespoons because it's easy to guesstimate a teaspoon from either amount. If you carry more than that, you can use standard cutlery at work to help you measure it out. But bringing a smaller but measured quantity of chia seeds cuts out the need for using a spoon to measure it out. You could keep a zipper-lock bag with the amount of chia you wish to consume in a day already measured out in it; that way, when the bag is empty, you'll know you've eaten all you need to!

You can also carry chia gel, but there are a couple issues to consider:

- **Refrigeration:** Letting chia gel get a bit warm is okay, but it might go bad if you leave it out for too long. It also has a better taste and texture chilled, in our humble opinion.

- **People's reactions:** Adding chia seeds to your food is a bit odd but not that uncommon; people sprinkle wheat germ or nuts on food all the time. Chia gel, however, may be looked upon as strange by others.

These are issues that can simply be resolved by using chia seeds instead of chia gel. However, if you have refrigeration close by—and the possible thought of other's reactions doesn't affect your ability to stay on the diet—go ahead and use chia gel. It's all about what makes you most comfortable.

For lunch and dinner, whether you've made your own or are eating out, you can add 1 teaspoon of chia to different parts of your meal. However, if you limit yourself to 1 or 2 teaspoons of chia in one meal, you might fall behind on your desire to get in 1 tablespoon (if you weigh around 100 pounds) or up to 2 tablespoons (if you weigh more like 200 pounds) during a full day. If you decide to up your intake and have 1 tablespoon of chia with your meal, make sure you drink lots of water during or after the meal to help you hydrate the chia without feeling thirsty.

Keeping Your Focus

As we discussed in Chapter 9, adding chia to your diet isn't simply going to make you lose a ton of weight or instantly get healthy. In order to keep on track with your goals and get the full benefit of chia, you'll need to develop an awareness of both your body and what you eat.

Listening to Your Body

As you learned earlier in the book, chia forms a gel in your stomach that slows the absorption of food. This, in turn, sends a powerful signal to your body that you're full and can stop eating.

However, even a powerful signal isn't going to help you much if you don't listen to it. There are all sorts of habits and social pressures that most people face that make it difficult to eat according to what your body is feeling.

The way food is presented can influence your eating habits. People have mostly been taught—directly or by example—to finish the food that's served to them. It's far more common for people to finish everything in front of them than it is to leave anything uneaten.

For example, most fast food is full of calories, salt, sugar, and fat and often comes packaged as "value meals," which include more food than most people might normally eat in a single meal. It would be hugely sensible to just eat part of a typical combo meal and save some of it or just throw it away, but that's rarely what happens. Instead, people tend to polish off the burger, eat all of the fries, and sip every last drop of that soda.

Social pressures encourage overeating, too. When you're the guest, it's considered rude not to eat food that someone has prepared and served. Even in restaurants, where you would imagine people wouldn't take it personally, the tendency is to eat everything you order. The availability of tempting appetizers and delicious desserts helps make for a meal that's double or triple what you might have eaten at home.

If your daily diet is largely constrained by habit and social pressure—and not by what your body is telling you—adding 100 or 200 calories a day of anything (even a superfood) is going to make you gain weight.

Adding superfoods to your diet doesn't only mean getting more nutrition and overall goodness. It also means reducing some of the other food you eat.

 SEEDS OF CHANGE

You can also take a "top down" approach to curbing how much you eat. Just eat the way you used to, but cut all your portion sizes by 5 or 10 percent. Keep eating the same fast food, the same restaurant meals, and so on with other people and alone, but always leave a few bites uneaten.

You can curb this urge to overeat by listening to your body, not just while you're eating, but all the time. Don't go get a meal just because it's lunch time; wait until you're hungry. Don't get fast food or a pizza just because it's convenient; think about how you really feel after eating it.

With chia in your diet, you're likely to have fewer pangs of hunger and more energy to move and do things. If you're already in the habit of listening to your body, or if you can get more in the habit of doing so, chia will help you balance your calorie consumption and your activity level. Just don't assume you can add any food to the exact same routine you've always followed and get the full benefit.

Developing Food Awareness

Listening to your body when you decide what to eat sounds great—and it is great. But by itself, it's not enough.

There's a delay built into your system that keeps you from feeling full until about 15 minutes after you're actually full. This phenomenon has been observed scientifically many times. Scientists can only theorize about the reason for it, and their best guess is that people were built to overeat due to scarcity of food. So in this case, listening to your body may not always be accurate.

There are also a lot of other outside voices that can sometimes override what your body is telling. Advertisements are all over–on the radio, on television, in print, and online. You see fast-food restaurants with convenient drive-thru windows everywhere. If you go to a convenience store for a pack of gum, you're likely to see hot dogs, pizza, and soda, all ready for you to grab and go. And you may have people at work, at home, and at friends' houses offering you all sorts of attractive things to eat.

Part of embracing superfoods, including chia, includes taking a critical look at the rest of what you eat. Adding superfoods will help you get healthier, but you'll only get the full benefit if you also subtract something.

You may have developed some defensive habits—for instance, you probably never grab one of those convenience-store hot dogs, knowing the chances are good it's been under a heat lamp a very long time. But you have to go further.

The easiest and most productive way to subtract is to develop a skeptical attitude toward all those ads—and even to your well-meaning co-workers and friends. It can seem unfriendly and standoffish not to grab a donut, a slice of pizza, or a cookie that someone has gone to the trouble to make. However, you'll be better able to stick to your diet and be much healthier in the long run.

Curbing the Secondary Effects of Chia

As you add chia to your diet and hopefully learn to listen to your body better along the way, you'll naturally adjust your diet for how much chia and water you need daily. However, you can sometimes encounter problems as you try to figure those things out, such as energy crashes and bloating.

The watchword is "gradually." Add chia a little bit at a time—1 or 2 tablespoons a day to begin with—to give yourself the chance to get used to its effects, the vast majority of which are positive.

The Chia Energy Crash

One thing to watch out for when using chia in your diet is the "chia energy crash." It's a side effect of the beneficial impact that eating chia usually has on your appetite and energy levels.

When you include chia in your diet, the gel that chia forms in your stomach fills part of the space in it, digests gradually, and provides you with energy the whole time. The gel also slows the digestion of food and makes that a longer-lasting energy source, too. While the gel is in your stomach, you get kind of spoiled—not feeling as hungry or as low on energy as you might otherwise expect. But when the chia gel is fully digested, the feeling of hunger and lack of energy that returns can feel like something of a shock.

You can also get this crash if you get used to eating chia a couple of times a day and then stop. You might suddenly feel that the smaller meals you've grown accustomed to eating are no longer enough.

The only trick you need to know to avoid this modest crash is to eat both chia and other foods regularly in small meals. The combination of food and chia will help you feel consistently comfortable and energized.

To avoid a harder energy crash that could come with physical activity, eat a healthy meal with chia close to the time you exercise while still leaving a one-hour buffer. For really extended exercise (more than a couple of hours), eat a light meal, with chia and plenty of water, during a break.

Chia Bloat

The opposite concern from a chia energy crash is chia bloat. Chia bloat is caused by the way chia works in your system, the way your body works with regard to feeling full, and your established eating habits.

Basically, chia and the water you need along with it take up a lot of room in your stomach. Normally, this is great, because it means you don't have to eat as much, and so you can lose or maintain weight more easily.

However, this can present two difficulties. First, when you're hungry, you tend to eat what you're used to eating to get full. With chia, though, you need less. If you eat like you're used to doing, plus chia and water, you can end up uncomfortably full. Second, you may overeat because the food's readily available. This can lead to a delayed reaction to feeling full, especially if it's part of a restaurant meal or otherwise placed in front of you. Add chia and water to that, and you can feel overly full.

So your long-standing habits, plus the fullness delay, plus adding chia and water to your diet, can set you up to overfill your stomach (sometimes by quite a bit). This can make you quite uncomfortably full at the end of a meal.

So what can you do to lessen or even avoid chia bloat?

- Go for a walk or do some light exercise after a meal. This helps you burn energy, which can help relieve the bloated feeling.

- Watch your portion sizes. Learn to eat less when accompanying your meals with chia, and then eat less than that. Eventually you'll find proportion sizes that work.

- Make sure the foods you eat count nutritionally for optimal daily and long-term health. This means lots of fresh greens from the farmer's market and a near-absence of low-value foods, such as french fries and beer.

Thankfully, the bloated feeling isn't the same as eating a truly massive dinner with calories in the many hundreds, or even over a thousand; the feeling is significantly due to chia, which your body doesn't take many calories from, and water, which is blessedly calorie free.

As a matter of fact, with chia, I often eat two meals a day, plus perhaps a decent-sized snack, rather than my traditional three. I'm still working on getting the portion sizes on the full meals down from what I'd gotten used to, but this is actually a great problem to have, for my weight and for my long-term health.

The Least You Need to Know

- Chia is great with eggs or as an egg substitute in early-morning omelettes before work.
- To control your hunger throughout the day and avoid binging, make sure to carry healthy snacks.
- Through portion control and light exercise, you can avoid the chia energy crash and chia bloat.

Chia Seed Diet Meal Plans

To achieve a healthy weight loss of 1 to 2 pounds a week, you'll need to cut back on your caloric intake by 500 calories a day or more, which means you'll eat about 3,500 fewer calories a week.

That may seem like a huge undertaking, but with a little planning on your part, it can be easy to cut the necessary calories to achieve the weight loss you desire—with chia playing a big part.

In this chapter, we break down how chia makes dieting easier and provide you with two-week meal plans based on your caloric intake.

In This Chapter

- How chia can help you with your weight-loss goals
- Calculating the caloric intake you'll need to lose weight
- Two-week chia seed meal plans to meet your needs
- Adapting the meal plans and keeping track of your progress

Why Dieting Is Easier with Chia and Vice Versa

If you're like most people, you probably don't have a physically challenging life. Unlike our ancestors, people today don't really get out in nature and are rarely scared in a way that's physically challenging (such as being chased by a hungry leopard!).

That means mealtimes are one of the rare times when your senses actually get activated. In fact, we believe that part of the reason people eat so much is because it's one of the few things that really feels good. Having a slice of chocolate cake or polishing off a cheeseburger and fries can make you associate big portions of processed food with happiness.

Now tie this in with dieting. You might be dreading the small-seeming meals that are part of a diet. However, by adding chia seeds to your meal, you'll make the dieting process much easier. If you're already half full with chia seeds by the time you sit down to the meal, the portion won't feel so small, and you'll feel full and satisfied in the end. The chia gel effect—by eating chia gel directly or putting chia seeds in your food that then create a gel in your stomach—takes away an awful lot of the discomfort and frustration that can come with dieting.

In fact, dieting solves a weird problem many have once adding chia seeds to their diet—not having to each so much food! Chia can help you redefine portion sizes and keep you feeling fuller longer—even on "diet" foods.

And the benefit is mutual. Adding ¼ cup of chia gel to granola every morning doesn't make it look better, and the goal of eating less and being healthier over time can feel a bit vague and far away. However, by including chia as part of a diet plan, you have an immediate goal—losing weight—that works as a stepping stone to your long-term goal.

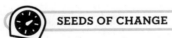 **SEEDS OF CHANGE**

> Some people say it takes about three weeks to establish a new habit; other people say it takes longer, even up to a year. Whatever the case, a couple weeks of dieting is a strong on-ramp to a long-term habit of incorporating chia into your food every day.

Subtracting the Fat: Calculating Your Weight-Loss Calorie Needs

To configure the chia seed diet to your needs, you first need to find out how many calories you can eat every day and lose weight. The next few sections walk you through the calculations to help you find out what you personally need.

Finding Your Basal Metabolic Rate

Let's start from the beginning and find out how many calories your body needs a day, or your basal metabolic rate (BMR). In order to do this, you first need to know your height in inches. If you don't know that number, here's an equation to help you:

Height in inches = (12 inches × number of feet) + remaining inches

Now plug your information into one of the following equations based on your gender:

Female: BMR = 655 + (4.35 × weight in pounds) + (4.7 × height in inches) − (4.7 × age in years)

Male: BMR = 66 + (6.23 × weight in pounds) + (12.7 × height in inches) − (6.8 × age in years)

For example, let's say you're a 40-year-old woman who weighs 145 pounds and is 5 feet 5 inches tall. First, you change your height from feet and inches to inches:

Height in inches = (12 inches × 5 feet) + 5 inches

Height in inches = 60 + 5 = 65 inches

Second, plug all your information into the equation for females to find out your BMR:

BMR = 655 + (4.35 × 145 pounds) + (4.7 × 65 inches) − (4.7 × 40 years of age)

BMR = 655 + (630.75) + (305.5) − (188)

BMR = 1,403.25 or 1,403 calories

So if you're a woman with these numbers, your base calories for the day are 1,403. This is what your body would need to function if you were to do absolutely nothing all day long except sit and breathe.

Finding Your Activity Factor

Now that you know how to calculate your BMR, you need to find out your "activity factor"—the number of calories you need to consume a day for healthy weight loss. This is based on the amount of exercise you get during the day. The following table shows you what calculation you should do based on your level of activity.

Activity Factor

Little to no exercise	Daily calories needed = BMR × 1.2
Light exercise (1 to 3 days per week)	Daily calories needed = BMR × 1.375
Moderate exercise (3 to 5 days per week)	Daily calories needed = BMR × 1.55
Heavy exercise (6 to 7 days per week)	Daily calories needed = BMR × 1.725
Very heavy exercise (twice per day; extra-heavy workouts)	Daily calories needed = BMR × 1.9

Let's use the information from the previous section as an example. You're the 40-year-old woman who needs 1,403 calories a day when at rest. If you exercise moderately—3 to 5 days a week for at least 30 minutes each time—here's the calculation you'd do to get your activity factor:

1,403 calories × 1.55 (moderate exercise) = 2,174.65 or 2,175 calories per day

This final number makes up the approximate total calories that your body needs to function each day.

Finding the Number of Calories You Need to Consume Daily

Once you've calculated the activity factor, you subtract 500 from that number to find the number of calories you need to consume daily for a healthy weight loss.

Using the example of the 40-year-old woman again:

2,175 calories per day − 500 calories = 1,675 calories a day

So if you had these numbers, you'd want to consume only 1,675 calories a day to lose weight. To help you plan your meals, you'd use the 1,500-calorie plan later in this chapter as the base.

You may think to yourself, "Hey, if I cut more than 500 calories, I will drop weight a lot faster!" This may be true, but if you cut too many calories, you run the risk of losing weight too quickly and then rebounding (which happens in many *fad diets*).

 DEFINITION

A **fad diet** is a diet designed to help you lose weight quickly that just happens to be popular at a given point in time. The problem with fad diets is they aren't always a healthy option, and rapid weight loss and taking in too little nutrition can cause you to rebound in your weight-loss attempt.

You also run the risk of your body going into starvation mode, which will cause your body to start holding onto unwanted fat (among other things) because it isn't being fed enough nutrients to keep it functioning optimally. Therefore, stay very close to the number you calculated to ensure you have a safe and healthy weight loss.

Two-Week Meal Plans for Your Calorie Needs

Now that you've calculated your daily caloric needs for weight loss, it's time to start using that number to lose weight.

The following tables provide two-week meal plans including chia for breakfast, lunch, and dinner (or "supper," depending on where you hail from). We've also added in snacks (because you've been so good all day!). These additions are strategic; having snacks is great for curbing your appetite between meals, which will help to eliminate any "binging" when you do sit down to a meal.

The meal plans are designed for 1,500- and 2,000-calorie diets. Your number probably won't exactly match 1,500 or 2,000, so just choose whichever one is closest to your target calories per day. These meal plans aren't concrete; you can change the meals as needed based on what foods you enjoy and your particular caloric needs. These are simply a blueprint to give you an idea of how you can incorporate chia into your diet successfully based on your weight-loss goals. To help you better manipulate the meal plans, we've included the calories for each meal so you can get an idea of where you can make adjustments. And if the meal plans you make up vary in calorie number—for example, one day has 1,534 calories and another has 1,478 calories—don't worry; you don't have to exactly match your number.

The meals in bold are ones for which you can find recipes in Part 4. For the other meals, you can find recipes for them on realsimple.com, cookinglight.com, bhg.com, eatingwell.com, and health.com; using the recipes in this book as examples, add chia seeds to them to bring them into the diet.

 CHIA CAUTION

Keep in mind that these meal plans don't include beverages. You should consume at least eight 8-ounce glasses of water a day, not including the extra water you should be consuming with the addition of the chia seeds in your diet (about 8 ounces of water per tablespoon). And be careful of high-calorie beverages, such as alcohol and fruit juice—you don't want to drink most of your calories.

Week 1 (1,500 Calories)

	Sunday	Monday	Tuesday	Wednesday	Thursday	Friday	Saturday
Breakfast	Blueberry-Banana Chia Smoothie (270 calories)	Ginger, Pumpkin, and Buckwheat Pancakes with Chia (240 calories)	Bear Naked Fruit and Nut Granola with Chia and 100-calorie Greek yogurt (255 calories)	Mango, Cacao Nibs, and Coconut Chia Smoothie (350 calories)	Chia-Cheddar Buckwheat Corn Muffins (330 calories)	Jamba Juice Apple-Cinnamon Yogurt with Chia and Bear Naked Fruit and Nut Granola with Chia (420 calories)	McDonald's Oatmeal with Chia (305 calories)
Lunch	Turkey hummus wrap, 1 handful (about 3 oz.) baked potato chips, and ½ cup cubed watermelon (458 calories)	Spicy Tortilla Vegetable Soup with Chia-Lime Sour Cream (440 calories)	Tuna pita sandwich and 1 handful (about 3 oz.) baked potato chips (449 calories)	Kale Caesar Salad with Parmesan-Chia-Hemp Crisps and 1 cup fresh blueberries (393 calories)	Veggie burger, 1 handful (about 3 oz.) baked potato chips, and ½ cup veggies of your choice (452 calories)	Napolitano Minestrone Soup with Chia (320 calories)	Pita pizza and a medium mixed green salad (about 1½ cups with 2 TB. low-fat dressing) (349 calories)
Afternoon Snack	15 almonds (150 calories)	¼ cup guacamole with 1 sliced medium bell pepper (150 calories)	Heirloom Tomato and Mozzarella Salad with Walnut-Chia-Basil Pesto (280 calories)	4 wheat melba crackers and 2 oz. herbed goat cheese (239 calories)	45 pistachios (148 calories)	Jamba Juice Pomegranate Smoothie with Chia (275 calories)	1 apple and 2 TB. peanut butter (304 calories)

	Sunday	Monday	Tuesday	Wednesday	Thursday	Friday	Saturday
Dinner	**Spaghetti Squash with Chia** (420 calories)	Roasted shrimp with roasted peppers and lemon (392 calories)	Chicken with sautéed spinach and mushrooms (295 calories)	**Chia Lasagna** (340 calories)	Crispy baked chicken (coated with corn flakes) and garlic collard greens (395 calories)	Pork tenderloin with cabbage and apple slaw (321 calories)	Grilled steak with roasted zucchini (321 calories)
Evening Snack	Tri-berry cobbler (162 calories)	**Chia Pudding** (290 calories)	Citrus angel cake (152 calories)	1 cup strawberries dipped in 1 TB. semisweet chocolate (115 calories)	2 oatmeal cookies (180 calories)	**Low-Fat Chia Chocolate Sorbet** (150 calories)	**Creamy Orange Chia Smoothie** (180 calories)
Total Calories for Day	1,460 calories	1,512 calories	1,431 calories	1,437 calories	1,505 calories	1,486 calories	1,459 calories

Week 2 (1,500 Calories)

	Sunday	Monday	Tuesday	Wednesday	Thursday	Friday	Saturday
Breakfast	Bear Naked Fruit and Nut Granola with Chia and 100-calorie Greek yogurt (255 calories)	McDonald's Oatmeal with Chia (305 calories)	Strawberry-Banana Chia Smoothie (substitute ¾ strawberries for blueberries in the recipe) (241 calories)	2 cups cantaloupe and 1 cup low-fat cottage cheese (300 calories)	Heirloom Tomato Frittata with Chia Seeds (200 calories)	Jamba Juice Apple-Cinnamon Yogurt with Chia and Bear Naked Fruit and Nut Granola with Chia (420 calories)	Chia and Egg in a "Whole" Avocado (410 calories)
Lunch	Chia Zucchini and Toasted Garlic Purée Soup with Parmesan and 8 crackers (380 calories)	Tomato and provolone sandwich with 1 handful (about 3 oz.) baked chips (499 calories)	Chia Greek Salad with Tuna and Honey-Lemon Vinaigrette (470 calories)	½ serving Spicy Tortilla Vegetable Soup with Chia-Lime Sour Cream and ½ serving Kale Caesar Salad with Parmesan-Chia-Hemp Crisps (375 calories)	Veggie burger, 1 handful (about 3 oz.) baked potato chips, and ½ cup veggies of your choice (452 calories)	Crab roll with 1 handful (about 3 oz.) baked potato chips (348 calories)	Chicken Waldorf salad over mixed greens (356 calories)
Afternoon Snack	1 cup grapes, 4 wheat Melba crackers, and 2 oz. herbed goat cheese (301 calories)	2 oatmeal cookies (180 calories)	45 pistachios (148 calories)	Carrots with Chia Greek Yogurt Dip (290 calories)	15 almonds (150 calories)	Chia-Cheddar Buckwheat Corn Muffins (330 calories)	1 apple and 2 TB. peanut butter (304 calories)

	Sunday	Monday	Tuesday	Wednesday	Thursday	Friday	Saturday
Dinner	Curried eggplant with tomatoes and basil (339 calories)	Chia Crab Imperial (350 calories)	Chicken with roasted sweet potato salad (388 calories)	Blackened salmon with broccoli rabe (339 calories)	Shrimp tacos with citrus cabbage slaw (392 calories)	Pork tenderloin with cabbage and apple slaw (321 calories)	Chia Stir-Fry Beef with Broccoli (250 calories)
Evening Snack	Caramel cream cheese custard (243 calories)	Low-Fat Chia Chocolate Sorbet (150 calories)	Old-fashioned fruit crumble (252 calories)	Creamy Orange Chia Smoothie (180 calories)	Chia Pudding (290 calories)	1 cup strawberries dipped in 1 TB. semisweet chocolate (115 calories)	Whoopie pies (202 calories)
Total Calories for Day	1,498 calories	1,484 calories	1,499 calories	1,484 calories	1,480 calories	1,534 calories	1,522 calories

Week 1 (2,000 Calories)

	Sunday	Monday	Tuesday	Wednesday	Thursday	Friday	Saturday
Breakfast	Blueberry-Banana Chia Smoothie (270 calories)	Ginger, Pumpkin, and Buckwheat Pancakes with Chia and 2 cooked eggs (430 calories)	Bear Naked Fruit and Nut Granola with Chia, 100-calorie Greek yogurt, and 1cup fresh blueberries (338 calories)	Mango, Cacao Nibs, and Coconut Chia Smoothie and 1 banana (455 calories)	Chia-Cheddar Buckwheat Corn Muffins (330 calories)	Jamba Juice Apple-Cinnamon Yogurt with Chia and Bear Naked Fruit and Nut Granola with Chia (420 calories)	McDonald's Oatmeal with Chia and 1 banana (410 calories)
Morning Snack	Chia and Hempseed Kale Chips (250 calories)	200-calorie granola bar of choice	1 cup fresh grapes and 1 serving (about 3 oz.) sharp cheddar cheese (203 calories)	1 handful (about 3 oz.) trail mix (225 calories)	200-calorie granola bar of choice	Carrots with Chia Greek Yogurt Dip (290 calories)	1 banana and 2 TB. peanut butter (288 calories)
Lunch	Turkey hummus wrap, 1 handful (about 3 oz.) baked potato chips, and 1/2 cup cubed watermelon (458 calories)	Spicy Tortilla Vegetable Soup with Chia-Lime Sour Cream (440 calories)	Tuna pita sandwich and 1 handful (about 3 oz.) baked potato chips (449 calories)	Kale Caesar Salad with Parmesan-Chia-Hemp Crisps and 1 cup fresh blueberries (393 calories)	Veggie burger, 1 handful (about 3 oz.) baked potato chips, 1/2 cup veggies of your choice, and 1 apple (568 calories)	Napolitano Minestrone Soup with Chia (320 calories)	Pita pizza and a medium mixed green salad (about 1 1/2 cups with 2 TB. low-fat dressing) (349 calories)

	Sunday	Monday	Tuesday	Wednesday	Thursday	Friday	Saturday
Afternoon Snack	15 almonds and 1 apple (266 calories)	¼ cup guacamole with 1 sliced medium bell pepper (150 calories)	**Heirloom Tomato and Mozzarella Salad with Walnut-Chia-Basil Pesto** and 1 (6-inch) whole-wheat pita (410 calories)	4 wheat Melba crackers and 2 oz. herbed goat cheese (239 calories)	45 pistachios (148 calories)	**Jamba Juice Pomegranate Smoothie with Chia** (275 calories)	1 medium apple and 2 TB. peanut butter (304 calories)
Dinner	Turkey meatloaf with mashed potatoes and 1 cup sautéed spinach (406 calories)	**Beef and Chia Stroganoff** (400 calories)	Chicken with sautéed spinach and mushrooms (295 calories)	Gnocchi with roasted vegetables (331 calories)	Crispy baked chicken (coated with corn flakes) and garlic collard greens (395 calories)	**Black Bean, Hemp, and Chia Patties** (410 calories)	Grilled steak with roasted zucchini and 1 whole-grain dinner roll (412 calories)
Evening Snack	Tri-berry cobbler and ¹/₂ cup frozen yogurt (279 calories)	**Chia Pudding** (290 calories)	Citrus angel cake, ¹/₂ cup frozen yogurt, and 1 cup sliced strawberries (321 calories)	1 cup strawberries dipped in 1 TB. semisweet chocolate and 2 oatmeal cookies (295 calories)	Chocolate decadence (315 calories)	Chocolate sherbet and 1 cup raspberries (215 calories)	**Creamy Orange Chia Smoothie** (180 calories)
Total Calories for Day	1,929 calories	1,910 calories	2,016 calories	1,938 calories	1,956 calories	1,930 calories	1,943 calories

Week 2 (2,000 Calories)

	Sunday	Monday	Tuesday	Wednesday	Thursday	Friday	Saturday
Breakfast	Bear Naked Fruit and Nut Granola with Chia, 1 cup fresh strawberries, and 100-calorie Greek yogurt (307 calories)	McDonald's Oatmeal with Chia (305 calories)	Strawberry-Banana Chia Smoothie (substitute ¾ strawberries for blueberries in the recipe) (241 calories)	2 cups cantaloupe, 1 cup low-fat cottage cheese, and 2 pieces whole-wheat toast (438 calories)	Heirloom Tomato Frittata with Chia Seeds and 2 slices whole-wheat toast (338 calories)	Jamba Juice Apple-Cinnamon Yogurt with Chia and Bear Naked Fruit and Nut Granola with Chia (420 calories)	Chia and Egg in a "Whole" Avocado (410 calories)
Morning Snack	200-calorie granola bar of choice and 1 cup fresh pineapple (278 calories)	1½ servings (about 5 oz.) trail mix (337 calories)	Chia Green Salad (240 calories)	1 handful (about 3 oz.) trail mix (225 calories)	1 cup fresh grapes and 1 serving (about 3 oz.) sharp cheddar cheese (203 calories)	Carrots with Chia Greek Yogurt Dip (290 calories)	1 cup fresh fruit and 1 cup low-fat cottage cheese (292 calories)
Lunch	Chia Zucchini and Toasted Garlic Purée Soup with Parmesan and 8 crackers (380 calories)	Tomato and provolone sandwich with 1 handful (about 3 oz.) baked chips (499 calories)	Chia Greek Salad with Tuna and Honey-Lemon Vinaigrette and 1 whole-wheat roll (584 calories)	½ serving Spicy Tortilla Vegetable Soup with Chia-Lime Sour Cream and ½ serving Kale Caesar Salad with Parmesan-Chia-Hemp Crisps (375 calories)	Veggie burger, 1 handful (about 3 oz.) baked potato chips, and ½ cup veggies of your choice (452 calories)	Crab roll with 1 handful (about 3 oz.) baked potato chips (348 calories)	Chicken Waldorf salad over mixed greens (356 calories)

	Sunday	Monday	Tuesday	Wednesday	Thursday	Friday	Saturday
Afternoon Snack	1 cup grapes, 4 wheat Melba crackers, and 2 oz. herbed goat cheese (301 calories)	2 oatmeal cookies (180 calories)	45 pistachios (148 calories)	½ cup guacamole with 1 handful (about 3 oz.) baked tortilla chips (286 calories)	15 almonds (150 calories)	**Chia-Cheddar Buckwheat Corn Muffins** and 2 cups fresh cantaloupe (452 calories)	**Chia Zucchini and Toasted Garlic Purée Soup with Parmesan** (220 calories)
Dinner	Curried eggplant with tomatoes and basil and 1 whole-wheat dinner roll (486 calories)	Roast beef salad with goat cheese and balsamic vinaigrette and 1 whole-wheat dinner roll (464 calories)	**Baked Ziti with Chia and Ricotta Cheese** (430 calories)	Blackened salmon with broccoli rabe and 1 medium baked potato (468 calories)	**Almond and Chia-Encrusted Chicken Breast** (380 calories)	Pork tenderloin with cabbage and apple slaw (321 calories)	Baked halibut with sugar snap pea salad and 1 cup wild rice (479 calories)
Evening Snack	Caramel cream cheese custard (243 calories)	Chocolate sherbet and 1 cup raspberries (215 calories)	**3 Chia Pizzelles** (360 calories)	**Creamy Orange Chia Smoothie** (180 calories)	**Chia Pudding** and 1 cup fresh raspberries (354 calories)	1 cup strawberries dipped in 1 TB. semisweet chocolate (115 calories)	Whoopie pies (202 calories)
Total Calories for Day	1,945 calories	2,000 calories	2,003 calories	1,992 calories	2,012 calories	1,944 calories	1,959 calories

Adapting the Meal Plans to Fit Your Preferences and Lifestyle

As we said before, the meal plans are only meant to give you an idea of what a day in that calorie level diet can look like. The use of chia in your daily diet will vary, but keep working to include it. We find the most important meal to include chia in each day is breakfast. Once you do that, a teaspoon of chia in a drink, plus a teaspoon or two in a meal, will get you a full supply of chia for that day. If you want to work up your own menu plan, just do some research on your favorite foods, their portion sizes, and the calories in each of the foods and then jot them down in a table similar to the ones we provided. It may take a little time to work out the calories properly, but getting personally involved in this way will help when it comes to achieving your weight-loss goals!

SEEDS OF CHANGE

For those of you who enjoy a little extra physical activity—I am using the term "enjoy" *very* loosely—be sure to subtract the calories you burned from the calories that you consumed so you have a more accurate picture of the calories you have taken in during the day.

It's also a good idea to keep a journal of some sort and record your meals and calories for each day, not forgetting to add in the calories for any beverages you consume. You can even record any physical activity you've done that day (including how you feel afterward).

You may need to add in a snack before and even after you work out if it helps you keep up your energy. However, including chia in the meals you eat early in the day will reduce your need for this kind of snacking.

The Least You Need to Know

- To find out what chia meal plan works best for you, calculate your BMR and activity factor. Subtract 500 from the activity factor, and you'll have an estimate of how many calories you can consume a day to lose weight.
- The two-week meal plans for the chia seed diet aren't set in stone. Feel free to make your own!
- Consume at least eight 8-ounce glasses of water a day, not including the water you should drink after consuming chia.
- Keeping a journal as you progress through the chia seed diet can help you track what and how much you're consuming throughout the day.

PART 4

Chia Recipes

This part provides chia recipes in every category—breakfast, lunch, and dinner; soups, salads, and snacks; and even sweet and savory desserts.

Chia recipes serve many purposes at the same time. The first purpose is obvious: When you're shopping or planning a meal or snack, you can look at the recipes in this part and find one that fits. This purpose alone is a "go-to" function for this book.

But wait, there's more. Even we don't think you're going to eat every meal from here on out from this part of the book. But after cooking specific dishes with chia, you learn how to combine chia with other ingredients and find out what you like or can at least tolerate.

Like a classically trained musician, using the recipes in this part is a worthwhile endeavor on its own, but the recipes also help you learn to do what the true masters do: improvise. By cooking the recipes here, you can get ideas for how to incorporate chia into almost anything you cook—and almost anything others cook for you.

Chia Addition Recipes

One of the great positives for a chia seed diet is that you can, in theory, just toss some chia seeds into almost any dish and enjoy it; the taste will be unchanged.

This is true, as far as it goes. Chia seeds have almost no taste. The flavor of foods with chia seeds added is almost identical to the flavor of foods without chia seeds added. However, there are a couple things to consider whenever you add chia to food that affect what happens when you add chia to existing recipes, as described here, and when you make recipes expressly designed to include chia (as you'll see in subsequent chapters).

A teaspoon of chia wants to absorb about 10 times its volume in water—that is, 10 teaspoons of water, which is just over three tablespoons, or nearly ¼ cup—and form the desirable chia gel in your stomach. If you add chia seeds to a recipe that doesn't have water in it and eat the resulting food, chia will try to get the water from other tissues in your body. If you drink lots of water at the same time, about a quarter cup of it will "feed" the chia, and you'll feel fine. However, if you add chia seeds to a "dry" recipe and don't drink water along with the food, you'll feel very thirsty indeed, somewhat out of proportion to the amount of water needed. That may involve drinking two or three 8-ounce glasses of water to offset the results of a "dry" recipe with chia added to it.

For instance, it's lots of fun and very nutritious to add 1 tablespoon chia to a couple of eggs in fixing various kinds of breakfasts. To help alleviate some thirst, you can also add a few extra tablespoons of milk to support chia's tendency to soak up liquids and form a gel. However, you should also make sure to drink a couple full glasses of water before, during, and after breakfast to meet your body's need for water after you have chia.

It's easier to add chia to a recipe in the form of chia gel (see Chapter 6 for how to make chia gel). Because chia gel already has water incorporated into it, it goes into your stomach and starts slowing your absorption of sugars and other sources of calories from food right away.

The bad news about chia gel is that the gel can be offputting when combined with a lot of different foods. For instance, you can add $^1/_3$ cup chia gel to your daily granola. Even with other additions, such as fruit and yogurt, the granola is a pretty different dish with the chia gel in there.

The good news, though, is there's no need to worry about drinking extra water when you use chia gel. And whatever form you use to get chia into your food, you benefit throughout the whole day.

Another thing with chia—which you might particularly notice with chia addition recipes—is that it makes you more regular, in the digestive sense of the term. Our ancestors ate much more fiber than we do, and they had, to be blunt, much more frequent and larger bowel movements than we do.

When a person eats "extra" fiber, by modern standards, he's just making a partial return to human evolutionary norms. But even this partial return can seem like a strain if you're not used to it. If you get 1 to 2 tablespoons a day of chia (or any other useful type of fiber) into your diet, you're setting the stage for long-term health—and quite possibly some short-term discomfort, as you'll need to go to the toilet more than you might be used to. This change to your digestive process is likely to feel like a bit of a shock.

Therefore, as you use the chia addition recipes in this chapter, be aware of your body. Don't be afraid to take careful note of the effects of adding chia and to adjust your use of chia in ways that make sense for you. However, do keep adding chia to your diet in as many ways as you sensibly can; the benefits will continue to accrue for the rest of your life.

 FOOD FOR THOUGHT

All of the recipes in this chapter and the rest in this part are protean (they're also "protein," as chia is a good source of protein). By "protean," we mean they're flexible and adaptable. The recipes are great for following "by the book," but also for adapting as a source of ideas for just about everything you eat.

Healthy Chia "Fresca"

Chia Fresca is diluted fruit juice with chia. In this version, the tart taste of lime is combined with the tangy taste of pomegranate to make a fun and nutritious drink. And no added sugar is required!

Yield:	Prep time:	Serving size:	
10 glasses Fresca	7 minutes	1 glass Fresca	
Each serving has:			
15 calories	5 calories from fat	0 g total fat	0 g saturated fat
0 mg cholesterol	10 mg sodium	3 g carbohydrates	1 g fiber
1 g sugar	0 g protein	36 mg potassium	15 mg calcium

9 cups water

$^1/_2$ cup lime juice

$^1/_2$ cup pomegranate juice

1 TB. chia seeds

about 20 ice cubes

1. In a plastic container with a lid, combine water, lime juice, pomegranate juice, and chia seeds. Put on lid, and stir or shake vigorously.

2. Wait 5 minutes, and stir or shake again.

3. Add ice cubes to glasses, pour Fresca into them, and serve.

 SEEDS OF CHANGE

For chia Fresca, try lemon juice instead of lime juice or apple juice instead of pomegranate. If you don't have a sweet juice, such as pomegranate or apple, use two tart juices (such as lemon and lime) and add sugar or stevia to taste.

Chia Pudding

By using premade chia gel, you can put together a sweet treat like pudding very quickly. For this chia pudding, the somewhat bland taste of the chia-milk gel is enlivened by honey, banana, and a bit of salt. This recipe is very adaptable to whatever kind of milk and whatever kind of fruit you have on hand.

Yield:	Prep time:	Cook time:	Serving size:
2 bowls pudding	5 minutes	15 minutes	1 bowl pudding

Each serving has:			
290 calories	100 calories from fat	11 g total fat	3 g saturated fat
20 mg cholesterol	700 mg sodium	38 g carbohydrates	9 g fiber
23 g sugar	12 g protein	617 mg potassium	414 mg calcium

2 cups 2% milk	1 large banana, sliced
1²/₃ cups chia gel	¹/₂ tsp. sea salt
1 tsp. honey	

1. In a medium saucepan over medium-high heat, heat 2% milk until almost boiling. Turn off heat.

2. Whisk in chia gel.

3. On the stove, reheat on low heat for 3 to 4 minutes or until bubbles start to form.

4. Add banana slices, honey, and sea salt on top and serve.

 SEEDS OF CHANGE

You can heat the milk for a warm dish on cold days or let it cool before serving on warm days. And if you need to use sugar in your pudding, granulated coconut palm sugar is a good alternative to white cane sugar. Coconut palm sugar is a bit fibrous and has some vitamins and minerals, so it digests more slowly and is more nutritious than cane sugar.

Brown Rice with Chia

Brown rice has a slightly nutty taste and a rich texture. Adding chia seeds to it provides some extra nuttiness to the taste while doing little to change the texture. Serve this dish with extra water or other drinks, as the chia seeds want to absorb about $^1/_2$ cup water per person.

Yield:	Prep time:	Cook time:	Serving size:
6 cups rice	10 minutes	1 hour	1 cup rice

Each serving has:			
290 calories	60 calories from fat	7 g total fat	3 g saturated fat
10 mg cholesterol	780 mg sodium	50 g carbohydrates	4 g fiber
1 g sugar	6 g protein	146 mg potassium	45 mg calcium

2 cups brown rice

$3^1/_2$ cups water

2 TB. unsalted butter

2 tsp. sea salt

3 TB. chia seeds

1. Preheat the oven to 350°F.

2. In a 10-inch square baking dish, place brown rice.

3. In a covered saucepan over low heat, bring water, unsalted butter, and sea salt to a boil.

4. As soon as the water reaches a boil, carefully pour boiling mixture into the baking dish and stir to combine.

5. Cover the baking dish tightly with aluminum foil and bake for 1 hour. Remove from the oven and remove the foil from the baking dish.

6. Sprinkle rice with chia seeds, fluff rice and chia with a fork, and serve.

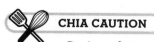 **CHIA CAUTION**

Don't use fast-cooking rice (10 minutes cooking time or less) for this recipe. Your body digests it very quickly, which means it gives you a blood sugar spike and doesn't exercise your digestive system like slow-cooked rice.

Baked Turkey Meatballs with Chia

Chia gel is sticky and therefore good for making meatballs hang together. The chia seeds add a slightly nutty flavor that complements the turkey well.

Yield:	Prep time:	Cook time:	Serving size:
16 meatballs	15 minutes	30 minutes	2 meatballs

Each serving has:			
120 calories	30 calories from fat	3.5 g total fat	0 g saturated fat
20 mg cholesterol	300 mg sodium	8 g carbohydrates	2 g fiber
3 g sugar	16 g protein	219 mg potassium	27 mg calcium

1 lb. 99% fat-free ground turkey	¹/₄ tsp. ground black pepper
³/₄ cup tomato paste	¹/₂ tsp. dry basil
³/₄ cup chia gel	¹/₂ tsp. granulated garlic
¹/₄ cup unseasoned breadcrumbs	1 TB. extra-virgin olive oil
¹/₄ tsp. sea salt	

1. Preheat the oven to 350°F.

2. In a large bowl, mix ground turkey, tomato paste, chia gel, unseasoned breadcrumbs, sea salt, black pepper, basil, garlic, and extra-virgin olive oil.

3. Scoop about 2 tablespoons mixture and roll to form into a meatball. Do the same with the rest of mixture. Place meatballs on a cookie sheet covered with aluminum foil.

4. Bake meatballs for 30 minutes. Meatballs should be brown and a bit shriveled when fully cooked. To be sure, cut one open and check it's no longer pink on inside.

5. Move meatballs to plates and serve.

 SEEDS OF CHANGE

Combine the meatballs with pasta sauce, brown rice (see the "Brown Rice with Chia" recipe in this chapter), and a vegetable or side salad for a complete meal.

Jamba Juice Pomegranate Smoothie with Chia

Adding chia to a smoothie is easy. You can add chia seeds to a smoothie you make yourself or just toss them into any existing smoothie—like one you get from Jamba Juice. Jamba Juice's pomegranate smoothie has the delicious, fruity taste of pomegranates, and better yet, it's good for you. Visit jambajuice.com for more information.

Yield:	Prep time:	Serving size:	
1 (16-ounce) smoothie	Varies with outlet and crowding	1 smoothie	
Each serving has:			
275 calories	10 calories from fat	1 g total fat	0 g saturated fat
5 mg cholesterol	35 mg sodium	62 g carbohydrates	4 g fiber
53 g sugar	3 g protein		99 mg calcium

1 (16-oz.) Jamba Juice Pomegranate Smoothie	1 tsp. chia seeds

1. Order Jamba Juice Pomegranate Smoothie.

2. Once you have it, add chia seeds and stir.

3. Eat.

 FOOD FOR THOUGHT

Many other restaurant smoothies or smoothies from small outlets use a lot of highly processed ingredients and sugar or other sweeteners. However, Jamba Juice is the largest chain that uses relatively fresh ingredients and offers an attractive range of healthy choices.

Bear Naked Fruit and Nut Granola with Chia

You can toss chia into all sorts of cereals and cereal mixes; it's especially nice in granola, as it makes little difference in the texture. This recipe uses Bear Naked Fruit and Nut Granola, a sweet and nutty granola you can find at any grocery store. Check out bearnaked.com for more information.

Yield:	Prep time:	Serving size:	
1 (about ¹/₄ cup) bowl granola	2 minutes	1 bowl granola	
Each serving has:			
155 calories	70 calories from fat	8 g total fat	1.5 g saturated fat
0 mg cholesterol	0 mg sodium	19 g carbohydrates	3 g fiber
6 g sugar	4 g protein	19 mg calcium	

¹/₄ cup Bear Naked Fruit and Nut Granola

¹/₄ cup chia gel

1. In a bowl, spoon Bear Naked Fruit and Nut Granola.

2. Add chia gel.

3. Eat.

 SEEDS OF CHANGE

Drink plenty of water when you add chia seeds to granola—about 3 ounces per teaspoon of chia, and then more to help you digest the granola. Drinking extra water to account for the chia seeds is not necessary when you use chia gel instead.

McDonald's Oatmeal with Chia

Not all of your meals are going to be cooked at home; sometimes, it's easier and faster to hit the drive-thru. But how do you avoid the sugar and fat and also add chia to your meal? Fear not; McDonald's oatmeal, with sweet maple and refreshing fruit, is a good option. By adding chia, you lower the glycemic index of the whole meal. Go to mcdonalds.com/us/en/food/food_quality/nutrition_choices.html for more information on nutrition options there.

Yield:	Prep time:	Cook time:	Serving size:
1 (1¼-cup) bowl oatmeal	Varies with outlet and crowding	1 bowl oatmeal	Varies with outlet and crowding

Each serving has:			
305 calories	45 calories from fat	5 g total fat	1.5 g saturated fat
5 mg cholesterol	160 mg sodium	59 g carbohydrates	6 g fiber
32 g sugar	6 g protein	29 mg calcium	

1 (1¼-cup) bowl McDonald's Fruit and Maple Oatmeal	1 tsp. chia seeds
	Water

1. Order McDonald's Fruit and Maple Oatmeal.

2. Once you have it, add chia seeds and stir. If necessary, add a few teaspoons of water to desired thickness.

3. Eat.

SEEDS OF CHANGE

To cut the thickening effect of chia in a dish like oatmeal, stir in a little milk, almond milk, or water.

Jamba Juice Apple-Cinnamon Yogurt with Chia

Frozen yogurt is a sweet treat with a smooth and creamy texture. It stands as an alternative to ice cream, which tends to be richer and have more calories and fat. Jamba Juice's tart and warm Apple-Cinnamon Yogurt is a good standard with which to begin experimenting. Visit jambajuice.com for more information on Jamba Juice frozen yogurt options.

Yield:	**Prep time:**	**Serving size:**	
1 (1/2-cup) frozen yogurt	Varies with outlet and crowding	1 frozen yogurt	
Each serving has:			
265 calories	13 calories from fat	4 g total fat	2 g saturated fat
10 mg cholesterol	150 mg sodium	55 g carbohydrates	7 g fiber
35 g sugar	9 g protein	49 mg calcium	

1 (1/2-cup) Jamba Juice Apple-Cinnamon Yogurt	1 tsp. chia seeds

1. Order Jamba Juice Apple-Cinnamon Yogurt.

2. Once you have it, add chia seeds, and stir.

3. Eat.

 FOOD FOR THOUGHT

You can easily add chia seeds or chia gel to any ice cream or frozen yogurt dish, as well as store-bought ice cream or frozen yogurt. To do this, combine the nutrition information on your chia package with the information available for your chosen yogurt or ice cream to come up with specific nutritional information for your own dish.

Drinks

One to 2 tablespoons of chia a day can be a pretty heavy lift until you get used to it, so adding chia to smoothies, milkshakes, teas, coffee, and kombucha—usually at the rate of about a teaspoon per serving—gives you an easier way to help yourself get there.

Chia in smoothies and milkshakes is a no-brainer for most of us. Both usually have various textures anyway, whether across different ones and or a single drink. Therefore, the slight "lumpiness" that goes with chia seeds shouldn't stand out too much.

Kombucha is fermented tea, a very healthy, refreshing drink that often has a tiny alcoholic kick. You may or may not be troubled by the added texture that chia adds to kombucha, but I think you'll find the kombucha recipe in this chapter to be quite nice.

Many people hold tea and coffee to be more or less sacred. Adding chia to your tea or coffee is likely to seem strange at first, but it's one way to get a fair amount of chia into your daily diet, combined with a drink that's warm and calming all on its own.

In This Chapter

- Refreshing fruit smoothies with chia
- Yummy chia milkshakes
- Chia lemonades and teas
- Amazing chia kombucha
- Enjoying chia in a cup of coffee

Try all of these drinks with an open mind, and if any work for you, you can incorporate them into your chia repertoire.

SEEDS OF CHANGE

We list honey as a sweetener for drinks in this chapter. However, if you're allergic or want an alternative that doesn't have actual sugar, try stevia. Stevia is a sweet herb about 40 times sweeter than sugar that's used to make a nonsugar sweetener. You can use fresh or dried stevia leaves directly.

Blueberry, Banana, and Chia Smoothie

This light smoothie, with sweet bananas and bright blueberries, can give you a delicious start to your day.

Yield:	Prep time:	Serving size:	
1 (10-oz.) smoothie	10 minutes	1 smoothie	
Each serving has:			
270 calories	60 calories from fat	7 g total fat	1 g saturated fat
0 mg cholesterol	125 mg sodium	49 g carbohydrates	8 g fiber
35 g sugar	7 g protein	189 mg potassium	534 mg calcium

4 TB. water	1 cup hemp milk
³/₄ cup frozen blueberries	1 TB. chia seeds
1 small banana	¹/₂ tsp. ground cinnamon
2 tsp. honey	

1. In a small bowl filled with water, soak chia seeds for 3 hours.

2. In a blender, place water with chia seeds, blueberries, banana, honey, and hemp milk, and blend on high speed until smooth.

3. Pour smoothie into a glass, sprinkle with cinnamon, and serve.

 SEEDS OF CHANGE

> Feel free to replace the hemp milk with almond milk, a different milk substitute, or dairy milk (low-fat or full-fat) to suit your dietary requirements and taste preferences. You can also freeze the banana to add more chill to the smoothie.

Mango, Cacao Nibs, and Coconut Smoothie with Chia

This smoothie features multiple flavors, such as sweet mango, fragrant coconut, and even a little chocolate. It's easy to add chia without disrupting the overall experience of drinking this smoothie, which could make it your go-to favorite for getting chia into your diet!

Yield:	Prep time:	Serving size:	
1 (10-oz.) smoothie	5 minutes	1 smoothie	

Each serving has:			
350 calories	150 calories from fat	16 g total fat	10 g saturated fat
0 mg cholesterol	5 mg sodium	49 g carbohydrates	8 g fiber
8 g sugar	3 g protein	22 mg potassium	44 mg calcium

1 cup fresh mango, diced

2 TB. mango nectar

1 TB. cacao nibs

2 TB. packaged or fresh unsweetened coconut flakes

2 tsp. chia seeds

1 to 2 ice cubes (optional)

1. In a blender, place mango, mango nectar, cacao nibs, unsweetened coconut flakes, chia seeds, and ice cubes (if using) and blend on the purée setting for 1 to 2 minutes until smooth.

2. Pour smoothie into a glass and serve.

Creamy Orange-Chia Smoothie

This classic smoothie with refreshing orange and creamy vanilla cream flavors is given a healthy chia twist.

Yield:	Prep time:	Serving size:	
1 (10-oz.) smoothie	5 minutes	1 smoothie	

Each serving has:			
180 calories	25 calories from fat	2.5 g total fat	0 g saturated fat
5 mg cholesterol	90 mg sodium	34 g carbohydrates	5 g fiber
22 g sugar	8 g protein	619 mg potassium	247 mg calcium

5 oz. frozen mandarin oranges	$1/4$ tsp. vanilla extract
$1/4$ cup orange juice	3 oz. plain nonfat yogurt
Zest of 1 orange	2 tsp. chia seeds

1. In a blender, place mandarin oranges, orange juice, orange zest, vanilla extract, plain nonfat yogurt, and chia seeds and blend on the purée setting for 1 to 2 minutes until smooth.

2. Pour smoothie into a glass and serve.

Nutty Banana-Chia Smoothie

This smoothie uses nuts as well as chia to add body and protein to a traditional banana-based smoothie.

Yield:	Prep time:	Serving size:	
1 (10-oz.) smoothie	10 minutes	1 smoothie	
Each serving has:			
490 calories	250 calories from fat	27 g total fat	3 g saturated fat
0 mg cholesterol	190 mg sodium	56 g carbohydrates	14 g fiber
27 g sugar	14 g protein	889 mg potassium	346 mg calcium

4 TB. water

1 TB. chia seeds

1 small banana

1 handful (about $^1/_4$ cup) unsalted peanuts

2 tsp. honey

1 cup almond milk

$^1/_2$ tsp. ground cinnamon

1. In a small bowl filled with water, soak chia seeds for 3 hours.

2. In a blender, place water with chia seeds, banana, peanuts, honey, and almond milk in a blender and blend on high speed until smooth.

3. Pour smoothie into a glass, sprinkle with cinnamon, and serve.

 SEEDS OF CHANGE

Feel free to replace almond milk with hemp milk, dairy milk (low-fat or full-fat), or a different milk substitute to suit your dietary requirements and taste preferences. You can also freeze the banana to add more chill to the smoothie.

Strawberry, Basil, and Chia Smoothie

Not many people think of putting basil in a smoothie, but I think you'll like it when you try it. The flavor of this smoothie is both unusual and refreshing, meshing both the sweetness of the strawberries with the slightly sweet flavor of the basil leaves.

Yield:	Prep time:	Serving size:	
1 (10-oz.) smoothie	5 minutes	1 smoothie	
Each serving has:			
140 calories	35 calories from fat	4 g total fat	1 g saturated fat
5 mg cholesterol	55 mg sodium	23 g carbohydrates	6 g fiber
15 g sugar	5 g protein	475 mg potassium	160 mg calcium

³/₄ cup fresh strawberries	5 leaves fresh basil
¹/₄ cup fresh or frozen strawberry juice	Dash (about ¹/₄ tsp.) aged balsamic vinegar
¹/₄ cup buttermilk	2 tsp. chia seeds

1. In a blender, place strawberries, strawberry juice, buttermilk, basil, aged balsamic vinegar, and chia seeds and blend on the purée setting for 1 to 2 minutes until smooth.

2. Pour smoothie into 2 glasses and serve.

 FOOD FOR THOUGHT

For a slightly different flavor, try using basil leaves as a substitute for mint leaves in desserts. You can also try basil leaves as a garnish and in drinks such as mojitos.

Peanut Butter, Banana, and Chia Smoothie

This smoothie combines smooth and creamy peanut butter with the fresh taste of bananas.

Yield:	Prep time:	Serving size:	
1 (10-oz.) smoothie	2 minutes	1 smoothie	
Each serving has:			
350 calories	130 calories from fat	14 g total fat	4.5 g saturated fat
5 mg cholesterol	470 mg sodium	24 g carbohydrates	4 g fiber
10 g sugar	34 g protein	192 mg potassium	141 mg calcium

$^1/_3$ banana

$1^1/_2$ TB. reduced-fat peanut butter

2 TB. fortified skim milk

1 oz. vanilla Greek yogurt

2 oz. silken tofu

2 TB. vanilla protein powder

1 tsp. chia seeds

$^1/_2$ cup ice

$^1/_4$ cup water

1. In a blender, combine banana, reduced-fat peanut butter, skim milk, vanilla Greek yogurt, silken tofu, vanilla protein powder, chia seeds, ice, and water and blend on high speed until smooth.

2. Pour into a glass and serve.

 FOOD FOR THOUGHT

You can get tofu in many different ways: flavored and unflavored, silken, firm, extra firm, and so on. For smoothies, silken tofu is preferred because of its smooth texture.

Morning Glory Chia Smoothie

This very colorful and tasty smoothie will surely get you rolling in the morning.

Yield:	Prep time:	Serving size:	
1 (10-oz.) smoothie	2 minutes	1 smoothie	

Each serving has:			
250 calories	30 calories from fat	3.5 g total fat	0 g saturated fat
0 mg cholesterol	260 mg sodium	28 g carbohydrates	7 g fiber
9 g sugar	28 g protein	307 mg potassium	109 mg calcium

6 TB. fortified orange juice

2 TB. strawberry protein powder

$1/3$ banana

3 oz. frozen berries of your choice, such as blackberries, raspberries, blueberries, and so on

3 oz. silken tofu

$1/4$ tsp. Splenda

1 tsp. chia seeds

$1/4$ cup ice

1. In a blender, combine fortified orange juice, strawberry protein powder, banana, frozen berries, silken tofu, Splenda, chia seeds, and ice and blend on high speed until smooth.

2. Pour into a glass and serve.

Pina Colada with Chia

Take a hiatus from your daily life with this Caribbean delight, which combines creamy Greek yogurt, sweet pineapple, and refreshing coconut milk.

Yield:	Prep time:	Serving size:	
1 (10-oz.) smoothie	2 minutes	1 smoothie	

Each serving has:			
210 calories	40 calories from fat	4.5 g total fat	3 g saturated fat
0 mg cholesterol	300 mg sodium	14 g carbohydrates	2 g fiber
9 g sugar	29 g protein	113 mg potassium	122 mg calcium

$^{1}/_{4}$ cup chopped pineapple

$^{1}/_{2}$ cup water

2 TB. fortified skim milk

$^{1}/_{4}$ cup light coconut milk

$^{1}/_{4}$ cup plain Greek yogurt

2 TB. plain protein powder

1 tsp. chia seeds

$^{1}/_{2}$ cup ice

1. In a blender, combine pineapple, water, skim milk, light coconut milk, Greek yogurt, protein powder, chia seeds, and ice and blend on high speed until smooth.

2. Pour into a glass and serve.

Frozen Banana-Chia Shake

Get the taste of a banana split with the nutrition of chia in this yummy shake.

Yield:	Prep time:	Serving size:	
1 (10-oz.) shake	2 minutes	1 shake	
Each serving has:			
260 calories	40 calories from fat	4.5 g total fat	2.5 g saturated fat
5 mg cholesterol	320 mg sodium	28 g carbohydrates	3 g fiber
19 g sugar	27 g protein	295 mg potassium	178 mg calcium

$^1/_4$ cup fortified skim milk

2 TB. vanilla protein powder

$^1/_3$ banana, sliced and frozen

1 oz. vanilla Greek yogurt

$^1/_4$ cup ice

1 TB. chocolate syrup

1 tsp. chia seeds

$^3/_4$ cup water

1 TB. light whipped cream

1. In a blender, combine skim milk, vanilla protein powder, banana slices, vanilla Greek yogurt, ice, chocolate syrup, chia seeds, and water and blend on high speed until smooth.

2. Pour into a glass, top with light whipped cream, and serve.

Fuzzy Navel Chia Milkshake

This peaches-and-cream milkshake adds the nutritional punch of chia.

Yield:	Prep time:	Serving size:	
1 (10-oz.) milkshake	2 minutes	1 milkshake	

Each serving has:			
280 calories	60 calories from fat	6 g total fat	3.5 g saturated fat
35 mg cholesterol	300 mg sodium	27 g carbohydrates	2 g fiber
15 g sugar	30 g protein	186 mg potassium	177 mg calcium

¼ cup fresh peaches	2 TB. vanilla protein powder
¼ cup low-fat vanilla frozen yogurt	1 tsp. chia seeds
¼ cup orange juice	1 oz. ice
1 oz. vanilla Greek yogurt	¼ cup water

1. Peel and deseed peaches.

2. In a blender, combine low-fat vanilla frozen yogurt, peaches, orange juice, vanilla Greek yogurt, vanilla protein powder, chia seeds, ice, and water and blend on high speed until smooth.

3. Pour into a glass and serve.

Mixed Berry and Chia Milkshake

With mixed berries, creamy Greek yogurt, and soothing vanilla, this milkshake is "berry" delicious!

Yield:	Prep time:	Serving size:	
8 (8-oz.) milkshakes	2 minutes	1 milkshake	

Each serving has:			
190 calories	60 calories from fat	6 g total fat	4.5 g saturated fat
0 mg cholesterol	280 mg sodium	7 g carbohydrates	3 g fiber
4 g sugar	27 g protein	0 mg potassium	72 mg calcium

2 cups vanilla Greek yogurt

3 cups water

3 cups frozen mixed berries

1 tsp. chia seeds

1 cup vanilla protein powder

2 oz. silken tofu

1. In a blender, combine vanilla Greek yogurt, water, frozen mixed berries, chia seeds, vanilla protein powder, and silken tofu and blend on high speed until smooth.

2. Pour into a glass and serve.

Lavender-Chia Lemonade

Fresh lemonade and soothing lavender combine to make a drink perfect for a hot summer day.

Yield:	Prep time:	Serving size:	
2 (6-oz.) glasses	10 minutes	1 glass	
Each serving has:			
170 calories	10 calories from fat	1 g total fat	0 g saturated fat
0 mg cholesterol	5 mg sodium	43 g carbohydrates	2 g fiber
34 g sugar	1 g protein	139 mg potassium	30 mg calcium

$^3/_4$ cup water

4 TB. honey

2 tsp. dried lavender

Juice of 4 lemons (about 12 TB.)

Zest of 1 lemon

2 tsp. chia seeds

1. In a medium saucepan over medium-high heat, heat water to a simmer. Stir in honey.

2. Add lavender, remove from heat, and let sit uncovered until cool.

3. Strain to remove lavender, and add lemon juice, lemon zest, and chia seeds.

4. Pour lemonade into 2 glasses filled with ice and serve.

Lemon-Lime-Chia Drink

Here's a quick way to get a few teaspoons of chia seeds into your diet and fill in a gap between meals. The tart taste of lemon and the tangy taste of lime combine with chia to make a fun and hearty drink.

Yield:	**Prep time:**	**Serving size:**	
4 (8-oz.) glasses	15 minutes	1 glass	
Each serving has:			
60 calories	25 calories from fat	3 g total fat	0 g saturated fat
0 mg cholesterol	10 mg sodium	9 g carbohydrates	4 g fiber
1 g sugar	2 g protein	88 mg potassium	70 mg calcium

3 cups water

$^1/_2$ cup lemon juice

$^1/_2$ cup lime juice

4 TB. chia seeds

1. In a medium bowl or pitcher, combine water, lemon juice, and lime juice.

2. Add chia seeds and stir.

3. Place in the refrigerator and chill for 5 minutes. Stir.

4. Put back in the refrigerator for 5 minutes and stir again.

5. Pour into glasses and serve.

Blackberry-Makrut-Chia Limeade

Makrut leaves have a unique taste that's a lot like lime, but with a strong scent and a unique quality all their own. This drink combines chia and makrut to make a unique drink that you'll surely come to love.

Yield:	Prep time:	Serving size:
4 (8-oz.) glasses	15 minutes	1 glass

Each serving has:			
45 calories	25 calories from fat	3 g total fat	0 g saturated fat
0 mg cholesterol	10 mg sodium	4 g carbohydrates	4 g fiber
0 g sugar	2 g protein	15 mg potassium	66 mg calcium

4 cups water	4 TB. chia seeds
4 makrut leaves, finely chopped	

1. In a medium bowl or pitcher, combine water, makrut leaves, and chia seeds.

2. Place in the refrigerator and chill for 5 minutes. Stir.

3. Put back in the refrigerator for 5 minutes and stir again.

4. Remove makrut leaves and serve.

 CHIA CAUTION

From looking at discussions online and talking to a bartender or two, it seems anyone making a drink with makrut in it seems compelled to add some form of alcohol as well. You don't have to go there! If you do, be very careful, as the exotic flavor of makrut can screen the warning signs that might otherwise tell you when you're overindulging.

Mint Sun Tea with Chia

This tea, with cool peppermint and mild honey, is a tasty, relaxing drink. Sun tea famously takes time to "cook" in the sun, but you can set this up in the morning and have it ready by that evening—an admirably quick turnaround.

Yield:	Prep time:	Serving size:	
4 (6-oz.) glasses	1 day	1 glass	
Each serving has:			
45 calories	10 calories from fat	1 g total fat	0 g saturated fat
0 mg cholesterol	10 mg sodium	10 g carbohydrates	1 g fiber
8 g sugar	1 g protein	10 mg potassium	25 mg calcium

3 cups water	2 TB. honey
2 cups peppermint leaves	4 tsp. chia seeds

1. In a glass jar with a lid, place water, peppermint leaves, and honey.

2. Put on lid and set jar in sunlight for 1 day.

3. Stir in chia seeds, pour into glasses filled with ice, and serve.

 SEEDS OF CHANGE

You can substitute spearmint, chocolate mint, pineapple mint, or any other mint for the peppermint.

Ch-ch-ch-chai-a

Chai is to tea as sangria is to wine—a spiced, livelier version of the original. As such, tea has many flavors and textures, making it a perfect "host" for adding chia.

Yield:	Prep time:	Cook time:	Serving size:
4 (6-oz.) mugs	10 minutes	20 minutes	1 mug

Each serving has:			
170 calories	110 calories from fat	12 g total fat	7 g saturated fat
40 mg cholesterol	20 mg sodium	15 g carbohydrates	1 g fiber
12 g sugar	1 g protein	35 mg potassium	47 mg calcium

3 green cardamom pods, toasted

8 pink peppercorns (about $^1/_4$ tsp.) toasted

$^1/_2$ TB. anise seed

6 cloves

1 TB. Darjeeling tea

4 cups water

$^1/_2$ cinnamon stick

8 thin slices gingerroot

1 bay leaf

3 TB. honey

$^1/_2$ cup heavy cream

Pinch fresh nutmeg

4 tsp. chia seeds

1. In a small sauté pan over medium-low heat, toast cardamom pods, pink peppercorns, anise seed, and cloves.

2. Remove toasted spices and place them and Darjeeling tea in cheesecloth. Tie cheesecloth shut with a string.

3. In a small saucepan, add water, cinnamon stick, gingerroot, and bay leaf. Bring to a boil over medium-high heat and simmer for 5 minutes.

4. Add cheesecloth with toasted spices and Darjeeling tea to the saucepan and steep for 10 minutes.

5. Take out cheesecloth and, over medium-high heat, bring tea to a simmer again.

6. Add honey, heavy cream, and chia seeds and stir until all ingredients are combined.

7. Pour in mugs, grate nutmeg over top, and serve.

 SEEDS OF CHANGE

Chai is like a salad, subject to as many variations in ingredients and preparation as you can think of. Therefore, feel free to mix things up to create chai that's flavorful, interesting, and fun for you.

If you'd like a lighter chai, replace the heavy cream with whole milk or skim milk.

English Breakfast Tea with Chia

Robust English Breakfast tea is a revered tradition in many places, not just England. The texture is a bit different with chia, but it's definitely something you can get used to—and benefit from.

Yield:	Prep time:	Cook time:	Serving size:
2 (6-oz.) mugs	10 minutes	20 minutes	1 mug

Each serving has:			
25 calories	10 calories from fat	1 g total fat	0 g saturated fat
0 mg cholesterol	20 mg sodium	3 g carbohydrates	1 g fiber
2 g sugar	1 g protein	16 mg potassium	71 mg calcium

1 cup water	1¹/₂ tsp. chia seeds
2 tsp. English Breakfast tea	¹/₄ cup hemp milk

1. In a small saucepan over high heat, bring water to a boil.

2. Add English Breakfast tea and let steep for 5 to 7 minutes.

3. Pour tea into mugs through cheesecloth to strain. Add chia seeds and hemp milk and stir.

4. Serve.

 CHIA CAUTION

English breakfast tea is a centuries-old tradition that's nearly sacrosanct to some. However, your health and well-being are likely to benefit if you can see your way clear to adding chia to the mix.

Chia Kombucha

Kombucha is legendary to some and novel to others. Kombucha can be made from everything from weak tea to strong coffee. However, this is a "straight" kombucha, in which the taste of tea is still quite recognizable but includes a hearty and refreshing taste all its own.

Yield:	Prep time:	Cook time:	Serving size:
5 (6-oz.) glasses	10 days	10 minutes	1 glass

Each serving has:			
40 calories	0 calories from fat	.5 g total fat	0 g saturated fat
0 mg cholesterol	10 mg sodium	10 g carbohydrates	1 g fiber
8 g sugar	2 g protein	312 mg potassium	114 mg calcium

8 cups water	2 cups kombucha starter
1 TB. honey	1 kombucha *scoby* in kombucha
4 bags black tea	1 TB. chia seeds

1. In a small saucepan over high heat, bring water to a boil. Stir in honey.

2. Add black teabags, turn off heat, and allow to steep while water cools, about 2 hours.

3. Remove black teabags and stir in kombucha starter. Pour into a 2-quart jar and add kombucha scoby and 2 tablespoons kombucha from scoby.

4. Cover the mouth of the jar with several layers of cheesecloth and secure with a rubber band.

5. Place the jar away from sunlight and traffic (avoid jostling) and allow to ferment for up to 1 week, watching for a new scoby layer to form on top.

6. After scoby layer appears, taste 1 tablespoon daily for sweetness and tartness until taste is satisfactory.

7. Remove scoby and bottle kombucha in 12-ounce or similar bottles, such as empty bottles from store-bought kombucha. Store the bottles at room temperature, out of direct sunlight, for 1 to 3 days.

8. When carbonation appears optimal, add chia seeds. Drink immediately as desired and chill the remaining bottles in the refrigerator to stop carbonation.

9. Drink within 1 month.

 DEFINITION

Scoby is an acronym for "symbiotic colony of bacteria and yeast." The scoby is what you place in a sweetened tea to make kombucha.

Do-It-Yourself Pomegranate-Chia Kombucha

Much of the fun of kombucha is the unusual texture and taste. Make it in a hurry—and add nutrition to your diet—by adding chia seeds to sweet pomegranate juice.

Yield:	Prep time:	Serving size:	
1 (8-oz.) glass	5 minutes	1 glass	
Each serving has:			
130 calories	13 calories from fat	1.5 g total fat	0 g saturated fat
0 mg cholesterol	25 mg sodium	28 g carbohydrates	2 g fiber
23 g sugar	2 g protein	8 mg potassium	60 mg calcium

$^3/_4$ cup pomegranate juice $^1/_4$ cup chia gel

1. Pour pomegranate juice into a glass.

2. Add the chia gel and stir vigorously.

3. Serve.

 FOOD FOR THOUGHT

You can add $^1/_4$ cup of chia gel to any drink. The chia gel will make the drink thicker and more satisfying and add a healthy dose of nutrition and digestive goodness.

Quick Chia Gel Coffee

This is the acidic, rich-tasting brew you're used to but thickened by chia gel. Once you get used to the texture, this drink can meet a lot of your dietary and alertness needs at once.

Yield:	Cook time:	Serving size:	
1 (8-oz.) mug	10 minutes	1 mug	

Each serving has:			
150 calories	60 calories from fat	7 g total fat	1 g saturated fat
19 mg cholesterol	15 mg sodium	19 g carbohydrates	9 g fiber
0 g sugar	4 g protein	37 mg potassium	154 mg calcium

1 cup chia gel   1 TB. instant coffee

1. In a small saucepan over high heat, bring chia gel to a boil.

2. Stir in instant coffee and remove from heat.

3. Pour into a mug and serve.

 CHIA CAUTION

Don't run chia gel through any kind of coffeemaker with thin tubes, as the chia seeds could clog it up.

Breakfasts

Breakfast is really the most important meal of the day for starting out with a healthy dollop of chia seeds or chia gel. If you get chia in early, you'll benefit the whole rest of the day. This is, of course, because of the gel chia and water form in your stomach. Once you get it established, the gel will slow down the beginnings of hunger pangs and release energy into your system steadily for hours.

If you skip chia with your breakfast—or, worse yet, skip breakfast—you can be in a constant battle with low blood sugar levels and resulting hard-to-manage hunger. However, if you eat breakfast, despite not naturally feeling as hungry as you will later, you can actually put your body on a beneficial cycle—especially with chia. Studies have shown that people who eat breakfast are less likely to gain weight and more likely to be healthy. Chia only adds to the benefits that go with eating a good breakfast.

Use the recipes in this chapter when you have time to put in a little effort. When you don't, use the breakfast recipes in Chapter 12 or just toss in a tablespoon full of chia seeds or $^1/_3$ cup of chia gel to any healthy thing you have handy, and get off to a good start that way.

In This Chapter

- Filling chia oatmeals and cereal
- Chia egg dishes
- Chia hazelnut spread
- Pancakes, scones, and muffins with chia
- Delicious chia bacon

Chia Pumpkin-Pie Oatmeal

If you like pumpkin pie, you'll love this healthy and delicious oatmeal.

Yield:	Prep time:	Cook time:	Serving size:
1 bowl oatmeal	2 minutes	15 minutes	1 bowl oatmeal

Each serving has:			
240 calories	100 calories from fat	11 g total fat	3 g saturated fat
5 mg cholesterol	40 mg sodium	27 g carbohydrates	6 g fiber
6 g sugar	10 g protein	181 mg potassium	172 mg calcium

$^1/_4$ cup skim milk	1 tsp. chia seeds
6 TB. water	2 TB. canned pumpkin
$^1/_4$ cup instant oatmeal	2 TB. sliced almonds
$^1/_2$ tsp. ground cinnamon	1 TB. sugar-free maple syrup
$^1/_2$ tsp. ground nutmeg	1 oz. vanilla Greek yogurt

1. In a medium saucepan over medium heat, bring skim milk and water to a gentle boil.

2. Add instant oatmeal, cinnamon, and nutmeg. Reduce heat to low and simmer for 8 minutes or until desired consistency is reached.

3. Stir in chia seeds, pumpkin, almonds, sugar-free maple syrup, and vanilla Greek yogurt.

4. Bring ingredients back up to temperature, about 4 to 5 minutes. Spoon into a bowl and serve.

Chilled Mixed Berry and Walnut Oatmeal with Chia

You are going to love this tasty breakfast treat of crunch walnuts and a sweet and tart mix of blueberries, blackberries, and raspberries.

Yield:	Prep time:	Serving size:	
1 bowl oatmeal	2 minutes plus overnight	1 bowl oatmeal	

Each serving has:			
342 calories	101 calories from fat	11 g total fat	.5 g saturated fat
0 mg cholesterol	95 mg sodium	53 g carbohydrates	18 g fiber
12 g sugar	11 g protein	132 mg potassium	220 mg calcium

$^1/_2$ cup rolled oats	1 tsp. chia seeds
$^1/_4$ cup almond milk	$^1/_2$ oz. (or about 10) blueberries
$^1/_4$ cup water	$^1/_2$ oz. (or about 3) blackberries
$^1/_2$ tsp. ground cinnamon	$^1/_2$ oz. (or about 5) raspberries
1 tsp. Splenda	1 TB. walnuts

1. In a small bowl, combine rolled oats, almond milk, water, cinnamon, Splenda, and chia seeds.

2. Cover with plastic wrap, place in the refrigerator, and chill overnight.

3. Add blueberries, blackberries, raspberries, and walnuts and serve.

 FOOD FOR THOUGHT

There are many different kinds of "milk" out there, such as almond, soy, oat, goat, cow, and so on. In this recipe, almond milk is used because it's slightly sweeter than the other milks and gives a nice, nutty flavor to the oatmeal.

Chia Chai-Craisin Oatmeal

This oatmeal combines sweet chai, tart cranberries, and creamy vanilla.

Yield:	Prep time:	Cook time:	Serving size:
1 bowl oatmeal	2 minutes	2 minutes	1 bowl oatmeal
Each serving has:			
290 calories	45 calories from fat	4.5 g total fat	0 g saturated fat
0 mg cholesterol	310 mg sodium	35 g carbohydrates	6 g fiber
5 g sugar	29 g protein	76 mg potassium	107 mg calcium

$1/2$ cup instant oatmeal	1 tsp. chia seeds
2 tsp. chai instant mix	$1/4$ cup light vanilla soy milk
2 tsp. dried cranberries	$3/4$ cup water
2 tsp. Splenda	2 TB. vanilla protein powder

1. In a small, microwave-safe bowl, combine oatmeal, chai instant mix, dried cranberries, Splenda, chia seeds, light vanilla soy milk, water, and vanilla protein powder.

2. Place the bowl in the microwave and cook on high for 2 minutes.

3. Stir and serve.

Chia Walnut-Banana Oatmeal

Cool banana and crunchy walnuts combine with quick-cooking oats to make a tasty and nutritious oatmeal.

Yield:	Prep time:	Cook time:	Serving size:
1 bowl oatmeal	2 minutes	8 minutes	1 bowl oatmeal

Each serving has:			
360 calories	70 calories from fat	7 g total fat	0 g saturated fat
0 mg cholesterol	320 mg sodium	45 g carbohydrates	8 g fiber
9 g sugar	30 g protein	280 mg potassium	113 mg calcium

$^1/_4$ cup light vanilla soy milk	2 TB. vanilla protein powder
1 cup water	1 tsp. chia seeds
$^1/_2$ cup quick-cooking oats	$^1/_2$ tsp. ground cinnamon
$^1/_2$ banana, mashed	$^1/_4$ tsp. ground nutmeg
$1^1/_2$ tsp. sugar-free maple syrup	$1^1/_2$ tsp. toasted walnuts

1. In a medium saucepan over medium-high heat, heat soy milk and water until almost boiling.

2. Add quick-cooking oats and stir until creamy, about 1 to 2 minutes.

3. Remove the saucepan from heat and stir in mashed banana, sugar-free maple syrup, vanilla protein powder, chia seeds, cinnamon, and nutmeg.

4. Pour into a bowl, top with walnuts, and serve.

Hot and Creamy Wheat-Berry Cereal with Chia

This hot cereal with tart cranberries and sweet brown sugar is a great way to get your protein in the morning.

Yield:	Prep time:	Cook time:	Serving size:
1 bowl cereal	2 minutes	10 minutes	1 bowl cereal

Each serving has:			
330 calories	50 calories from fat	5 g total fat	0 g saturated fat
0 mg cholesterol	400 mg sodium	42 g carbohydrates	8 g fiber
6 g sugar	30 g protein	184 mg potassium	205 mg calcium

1 tsp. slivered almonds	$^1/_2$ tsp. brown sugar Splenda
$^1/_4$ cup plus 1 tsp. rolled oats	1 tsp. chia seeds
1 TB. dried cranberries	2 TB. vanilla protein powder
$^3/_4$ cup light vanilla soy milk	$^1/_2$ tsp. ground cinnamon
$^1/_4$ cup plus 1 tsp. cooked wheat berries	

1. In a small sauté pan over medium heat, toast almonds until you can smell them, about 5 minutes.

2. In a large, microwave-safe bowl, combine rolled oats, cranberries, and light vanilla soy milk.

3. Place the bowl in the microwave and microwave on high, uncovered, for 3 minutes.

4. Stir in cooked wheat berries and microwave again until hot, about 1 to 2 minutes.

5. Let oatmeal stand for 1 minute.

6. Stir in brown sugar Splenda, chia seeds, vanilla protein powder, and cinnamon.

7. Sprinkle with toasted almonds and serve.

 CHIA CAUTION

When toasting the almonds, make sure to move the pan quite often when it starts to get hot. Also, make sure you pay close attention to the almonds, because they will burn quickly. As soon as you smell that toasted almond aroma, remove the almonds from the pan.

Chia Scrambled Eggs

Eggs are replaced in this recipe, which has a spicy and nutritious twist on the typical morning staple.

Yield:	Prep time:	Cook time:	Serving size:
1 plate eggs	5 minutes	2 minutes	1 plate eggs
Each serving has:			
110 calories	60 calories from fat	7 g total fat	1 g saturated fat
0 mg cholesterol	730 mg sodium	2 g carbohydrates	1 g fiber
0 g sugar	10 g protein	120 mg potassium	103 mg calcium

3 oz. liquid egg substitute	$^1/_4$ tsp. sea salt
1 tsp. chia seeds	$^1/_4$ tsp. black pepper
1 tsp. ground turmeric	1 tsp. olive oil
$^1/_2$ tsp. hot pepper sauce	1 oz. firm tofu

1. In a small bowl, blend liquid egg substitute, chia seeds, turmeric, hot pepper sauce, sea salt and black pepper with a fork.

2. In a small nonstick skillet over medium-low heat, heat olive oil.

3. Add firm tofu to the pan and cook, stirring, until warmed through, about 20 to 30 seconds.

4. Add egg mixture and stir until the egg is set but still creamy, about 20 to 30 seconds.

5. Put onto a plate and serve immediately.

 FOOD FOR THOUGHT

Turmeric is a spice known as the "Indian saffron" because of its golden yellow color.

Chia and Egg in a "Whole" Avocado

The refreshing and fulfilling flavor of avocado and the rich flavor of baked eggs are a wonderful combination. When you add chia, the whole has an awful lot of the nutrition you need for your day.

Yield:	Prep time:	Cook time:	Serving size:
4 avocado halves and 4 tsp. chia and egg mix	10 minutes	15 minutes	2 avocado halves and 2 tsp. chia and egg mix

Each serving has:			
410 calories	300 calories from fat	33 g total fat	6 g saturated fat
435 mg cholesterol	140 mg sodium	18 g carbohydrates	6 g fiber
0 g sugar	19 g protein	724 mg potassium	82 mg calcium

2 ripe, fresh avocados	4 large eggs
4 tsp. queso fresco	Sea salt
1 tsp. chia seeds	Cracked black pepper
2 TB. fresh chives, chopped	

1. Preheat the oven to 350°F.

2. Slice avocados in half and remove pits. Scoop out about $1^1/_2$ to 2 tablespoons of avocado flesh and place hollowed halves in a small baking dish.

3. In a medium bowl, mix queso fresco, chia seeds, and chives. Place $1^1/_2$ teaspoons of mixture into the bottom of each avocado half.

4. Carefully crack 1 egg into each avocado half.

5. Place avocado halves on a cookie sheet covered with aluminum foil.

6. Put in the oven and bake for 15 to 20 minutes.

7. Remove from the oven, add sea salt and black pepper to taste, and serve with your favorite salsa or topping.

Turkey, Tomato, and Scallion Mini Quiches with Chia

Have some fun with breakfast with these mini quiches that combine turkey, tomatoes, and scallions.

Yield:	Prep time:	Cook time:	Serving size:
8 mini quiches	5 minutes	25 to 28 minutes	1 mini quiche

Each serving has:			
170 calories	70 calories from fat	7 g total fat	3.5 g saturated fat
30 mg cholesterol	230 mg sodium	6 g carbohydrates	1 g fiber
4 g sugar	19 g protein	305 mg potassium	368 mg calcium

$2^{1}/_{4}$ cups liquid egg substitute

1 tsp. chia seeds

1 cup skim milk

1 bunch (or about 6) scallions

$^{1}/_{2}$ cup tomato, diced

$1^{1}/_{2}$ cups shredded low-fat Swiss cheese

$^{1}/_{4}$ lb. cooked turkey, sliced into $^{1}/_{4}$-in. chunks

1 tsp. black pepper

1. Preheat the oven to 350°F.

2. Coat 12 nonstick muffin cups with cooking spray.

3. In a large bowl, whisk liquid egg substitute, chia seeds, and skim milk. Add scallions, diced tomato, low-fat Swiss cheese, turkey, and black pepper and stir to combine.

4. Divide egg mixture evenly among prepared muffin cups.

5. Place in the oven and bake until beginning to brown on top, about 25 to 28 minutes.

6. Run a knife around edges to loosen mini quiches from the cups, place on plates, and serve.

Spinach, Tomato, and Feta Omelette with Chia

This bright and colorful omelette with refreshing cherry tomatoes, peppery spinach, and creamy feta cheese is sure to please your taste buds.

Yield:	Prep time:	Cook time:	Serving size:
1 omelette	2 minutes	8 minutes	1 omelette

Each serving has:			
180 calories	70 calories from fat	8 g total fat	2 g saturated fat
5 mg cholesterol	770 mg sodium	10 g carbohydrates	4 g fiber
4 g sugar	18 g protein	471 mg potassium	180 mg calcium

1 tsp. olive oil	$^1/_8$ cup skim milk
5 cherry tomatoes	$^1/_2$ oz. low-fat feta cheese
1 scallion	Pinch sea salt
1 cup baby spinach	Pinch black pepper
5 oz. liquid egg substitute	1 TB. fresh basil, cut chiffonade
1 tsp. chia seeds	

1. Spray a small nonstick skillet with cooking spray. Add olive oil and heat over medium-high heat.

2. Dice cherry tomatoes small, slice scallion, and add both to sauté pan. Cook, stirring once or twice, until softened, about 1 to 2 minutes.

3. Place baby spinach on top, cover skillet, and let spinach wilt, about 30 seconds. Stir to combine.

4. In a small bowl, combine liquid egg substitute, chia seeds, and skim milk.

5. Pour egg mixture into the skillet. Reduce heat to medium-low and continue cooking, stirring constantly with a heatproof rubber spatula until the egg is starting to set, about 20 seconds.

6. Continue cooking, lifting edges so uncooked egg will flow underneath, until mostly set, about 30 more seconds.

7. Sprinkle low-fat feta cheese, sea salt, and black pepper over egg.

8. Cover, reduce heat to low and cook until egg is completely set and cheese is melted, about 2 minutes. Fold over using the spatula.

9. Place on a plate, garnish with basil, and serve.

DEFINITION

Chiffonade is the cutting of leafy vegetables such as herbs, spinach, and so on into thin strips. To do this, stack the leaves largest to smallest, roll tightly from stem to the tip of the leaf, and cut across the rolled leaves with a sharp knife, producing fine ribbons.

Cheesy Egg and Polenta Chia Casserole

This delicious omelet is bright and colorful and is sure to please your taste buds.

Yield:	Prep time:	Cook time:	Serving size:
8 squares casserole	5 minutes	40 to 45 minutes	1 square casserole

Each serving has:			
220 calories	70 calories from fat	8 g total fat	2 g saturated fat
20 mg cholesterol	610 mg sodium	20 g carbohydrates	1 g fiber
2 g sugar	15 g protein	101 mg potassium	197 mg calcium

1 TB. plus 2 tsp. olive oil

$^1/_3$ cup white onion

4 cups low-sodium and low-fat vegetable broth

1 cup yellow cornmeal

$^1/_2$ tsp. sea salt

$^1/_2$ tsp. black pepper

6 oz. Italian turkey sausage

$^1/_2$ cup reduced-fat mozzarella cheese

$^1/_2$ cup grated Parmesan cheese

$1^1/_2$ cups liquid egg substitute

1 tsp. chia seeds

1. In a large saucepan over medium heat, heat 1 tablespoon olive oil. Add white onion and cook, stirring, until softened but not browned, about 2 to 3 minutes.

2. Add vegetable broth and bring to a boil over medium-high heat.

3. Gradually whisk in yellow cornmeal and add sea salt and black pepper. Cook over medium heat, whisking constantly until polenta bubbles, about 1 to 2 minutes.

4. Reduce heat to low and cook, whisking frequently, until very thick, about 10 to 15 minutes.

5. In a large skillet over medium heat, heat remaining 2 teaspoons oil. Add Italian turkey sausage and cook, stirring and breaking sausage into small pieces with a spoon, until lightly browned and no longer pink, about 4 minutes.

6. Drain sausage if necessary and transfer to a cutting board to let cool. When cool enough to handle, finely chop sausage.

7. Position rack in upper third of the oven and preheat to 350°F. Coat a 9-by-13-inch baking pan with cooking spray.

8. Stir reduced-fat mozzarella cheese and ¼ cup Parmesan cheese in polenta mixture. If polenta seems too stiff, add small amounts of water to thin it to a thick but not stiff consistency. Spread polenta in the prepared pan.

9. Make six 2-inch-wide indentations in polenta with the back of a tablespoon. Fold liquid egg substitute and chia seeds into polenta.

10. Sprinkle sausage and remaining ¼ cup Parmesan evenly on top of polenta.

11. Place in the oven and bake for 15 minutes. Broil until egg is set, about 2 to 4 minutes.

12. Let casserole stand for 5 minutes. Serve.

Heirloom Tomato Frittata with Chia Seeds

This frittata is delicious and light, with fresh tomatoes, basil, and creamy cheddar cheese.

Yield:	Prep time:	Cook time:	Serving size:
1 frittata	10 minutes	18 to 22 minutes	$^1/_6$ frittata

Each serving has:			
200 calories	130 calories from fat	15 g total fat	3.5 g saturated fat
165 mg cholesterol	120 mg sodium	10 g carbohydrates	5 g fiber
3 g sugar	10 g protein	423 mg potassium	230 mg calcium

4 medium eggs	Cracked black pepper
$^1/_4$ cup reduced-fat cheddar cheese, shredded	2 TB. extra-virgin olive oil
3 TB. chia seeds	3 cloves garlic, chopped
$^3/_4$ cup water	1 lb. heirloom tomatoes, sliced
Sea salt	1 bunch basil leaves, torn

1. Preheat the oven to 375°F.

2. In a medium bowl, crack eggs and whisk together.

3. Add cheddar cheese, chia seeds, water, sea salt to taste, and black pepper to taste and whisk further.

4. In a medium saucepan on medium-low heat, add extra-virgin olive oil.

5. Add garlic and sauté until golden brown, about 8 to 10 minutes, stirring occasionally. Season with sea salt and black pepper to taste.

6. Add egg mixture, heirloom tomatoes, and $^1/_2$ of basil and mix.

7. Move the saucepan to the oven and bake for 10 to 12 minutes or until firm.

8. Put on plates, garnish with remaining $^1/_2$ of basil, and serve.

Fried Chia Matzoh

Matzoh's flavor can be kind of bland and bready, and people either love it or don't like it. This version adds the rich flavor of eggs plus chia and gives you the chance to experience matzoh in a new way.

Yield:	Prep time:	Cook time:	Serving size:
4 slices matzoh	10 minutes	25 minutes	1 slice matzoh

Each serving has:			
320 calories	170 calories from fat	19 g total fat	6 g saturated fat
230 mg cholesterol	110 mg sodium	27 g carbohydrates	2 g fiber
1 g sugar	10 g protein	54 mg potassium	52 mg calcium

4 sheets matzoh	Sea salt
4 large eggs	Ground black pepper
2 TB. chia seeds	2 TB. butter
½ cup water	2 TB. extra-virgin olive oil

1. In a medium pot filled with cold water, soak matzoh for 2 minutes.

2. Drain well and break matzoh into medium-size pieces.

3. In a small bowl, add chia seeds and water and mix. Add eggs, sea salt to taste, and black pepper to taste and whisk.

4. In a medium sauté pan over medium heat, heat up butter and extra-virgin olive oil.

5. Add matzoh evenly in pan and pour egg mixture over top.

6. Cook on one side until golden brown, about 10 minutes. Gently flip over with a spatula to cook the other side until golden brown, about 10 minutes.

7. Put on plates and serve with fresh fruit jam or your favorite topping.

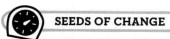 **SEEDS OF CHANGE**

Get the best and most authentic matzoh you can find for this recipe. The simplicity of this recipe will allow the flavor of high-quality matzoh to shine through.

Chia Hazelnut Spread

Known commonly by the brand name Nutella, the flavor of hazelnut spread is a favorite among vegans and other health-conscious people. It's sweet and delicious in its own right, with both a nutty and chocolatey taste and a great substitute for other, less healthy sweets. This version makes a great host flavor and spread for adding more chia into your diet.

Yield:	Prep time:	Cook time:	Serving size:
6 TB. spread	20 minutes	2 to 3 minutes	about 1^1/$_2$ TB. spread
Each serving has:			
320 calories	210 calories from fat	23 g total fat	12 g saturated fat
25 mg cholesterol	5 mg sodium	25 g carbohydrates	5 g fiber
15 g sugar	5 g protein	128 mg potassium	50 mg calcium

^{1}/$_4$ cup raw cashews

^{1}/$_4$ cup dried unsweetened coconut

2 TB. cacao nips

^{1}/$_3$ cup maple syrup

2 TB. extra-virgin coconut oil

2 TB. maca powder

3 TB. chia seeds

2 tsp. vanilla extract

Sea salt

1. Preheat the oven to 375°F.

2. On a sheet pan, place cashews. Place in the oven and roast for 2 to 3 minutes until lightly browned.

3. In a food processor, place roasted cashews, unsweetened coconut, cacao nips, maple syrup, extra-virgin coconut oil, maca powder, chia seeds, vanilla extract, and sea salt to taste and purée until smooth.

4. Serve spread on your favorite crepes, breads, muffins, or pastries.

Blackberry-Ricotta Pancakes with Chia

Ricotta pancakes get a tart twist with the addition of blackberries in this yummy breakfast food.

Yield:	Prep time:	Cook time:	Serving size:
16 pancakes	5 minutes	10 minutes	2 pancakes

Each serving has:			
200 calories	50 calories from fat	6 g total fat	2.5 g saturated fat
10 mg cholesterol	360 mg sodium	24 g carbohydrates	4 g fiber
5 g sugar	13 g protein	121 mg potassium	199 mg calcium

1 cup whole-wheat flour	³/₄ cup part-skim ricotta cheese
¹/₄ cup plus 4 TB. all-purpose flour	³/₄ cup vanilla Greek yogurt
¹/₄ cup vanilla protein powder	³/₄ cup liquid egg substitute
2 tsp. Splenda	1 cup fat-free buttermilk
1 tsp. chia seeds	2 tsp. lemon zest
2 tsp. baking powder	2 TB. lemon juice
¹/₂ tsp. baking soda	3 tsp. vegetable oil
1 tsp. ground nutmeg	1¹/₂ cups frozen blackberries

1. In a small bowl, combine whole-wheat flour, all-purpose flour, vanilla protein powder, Splenda, chia seeds, baking powder, baking soda, and nutmeg.

2. In a large bowl, whisk part-skim ricotta cheese, vanilla Greek yogurt, liquid egg substitute, fat-free buttermilk, lemon zest, and lemon juice until smooth.

3. Add dry ingredients to wet ingredients and stir until just combined.

4. Brush a large nonstick skillet with vegetable oil and heat over medium heat until hot.

5. Using a generous ¼ cup batter for each pancake, pour the batter for 2 pancakes into the pan, sprinkle about ⅛ cup blackberries between each, and cook until edges are dry and bubbles begin to form, about 2 minutes.

6. Flip pancakes and cook until golden brown, about 2 more minutes. Repeat with remaining batter and blackberries, adjusting the heat as necessary to prevent burning.

7. Place pancakes on plates and serve.

 SEEDS OF CHANGE

Greek yogurt, which is used in this recipe, is preferred because it's higher in protein than regular yogurt. Feel free to swap in a fat-free or reduced-fat version.

Ginger, Pumpkin, and Buckwheat Pancakes with Chia

These delicious pancakes are great for fall, with hints of zesty ginger, creamy pumpkin, and nutty buckwheat in the mix!

Yield:	Prep time:	Cook time:	Serving size:
12 pancakes	15 minutes	20 minutes	3 pancakes

Each serving has:			
240 calories	130 calories from fat	15 g total fat	3.5 g saturated fat
325 mg cholesterol	260 mg sodium	13 g carbohydrates	6 g fiber
2 g sugar	14 g protein	81 mg potassium	101 mg calcium

$^1/_3$ cup buckwheat flour

$^1/_4$ cup almond flour

Pinch sea salt

$^1/_2$ tsp. baking soda

1 tsp. ground cinnamon

3 TB. chia seeds

1 tsp. ground ginger

$^1/_4$ tsp. ground nutmeg

6 large eggs

$^1/_3$ cup canned pumpkin purée

1 tsp. vanilla extract

$^1/_4$ cup whole milk or your favorite nondairy replacement

$^1/_2$ tsp. coconut oil

1. In a medium bowl, place buckwheat flour, almond flour, sea salt, baking soda, cinnamon, chia seeds, ginger, and nutmeg.

2. Add eggs, pumpkin purée, vanilla extract, and whole milk and blend together with a whisk or hand mixer until a smooth batter is formed.

3. In a medium skillet over medium heat, add coconut oil to grease the pan.

4. Add ¼-cup scoop of batter to the pan and cook until golden brown on edges and bubbles appear on top, about 2 minutes.

5. Flip over and cook for 2 more minutes, adding more coconut oil if necessary. Repeat with remaining batter.

6. Place pancakes on plates and serve with butter or almond butter and syrup.

CHIA CAUTION

Pancakes tend to swell in your stomach and leave you feeling bloated after eating. Chia seeds or chia gel can also swell in your stomach and leave you feeling bloated after eating. You can see where I'm going with this. Eat chia pancakes in a very moderate fashion, and take a break of 10 minutes or so after eating each pancake. The cooking and serving process may impose this kind of pause on you already, though, especially if you're sharing.

Black Sesame Rice Flour and Chia Crepe

This is a bready food that can serve as a nutritious alternative to mainstream breads. This can be a rich and delicious substitute for pancakes.

Yield:	Prep time:	Cook time:	Serving size:
8 crepes	50 minutes	25 minutes	2 crepes

Each serving has:			
300 calories	80 calories from fat	9 g total fat	3.5 g saturated fat
120 mg cholesterol	240 mg sodium	46 g carbohydrates	2 g fiber
13 g sugar	9 g protein	168 mg potassium	143 mg calcium

$^1/_4$ tsp. sea salt	2 large eggs
$1^1/_2$ cups 2% milk	2 tsp. vanilla extract
3 TB. honey	1 TB. chia seeds
1 cup rice flour	$^1/_2$ TB. black sesame seeds
1 TB. butter, melted	Coconut oil

1. In a blender, place sea salt, 2% milk, honey, rice flour, butter, eggs, and vanilla extract and blend on slow speed until smooth.

2. Let crepe batter rest for 20 minutes.

3. Stir in chia seeds and black sesame seeds and blend on slow speed until smooth.

4. Let crepe batter rest for 30 minutes.

5. Heat a crepe pan or medium saucepan over low to medium heat.

6. Add enough coconut oil to coat the pan and add ⅛ cup crepe batter.

7. Let batter cover entire bottom of the pan by swirling it to coat evenly and cook on one side until set and bubbles form on the top, about 1 minute 30 seconds.

8. Flip over and finish cooking other side, about 1 minute 30 seconds. Repeat the process with remaining crepe batter.

9. Put crepes on plates and serve.

Chia Cheddar-Buckwheat Corn Muffins

Corn muffins with buckwheat have a rich and savory flavor. They're a great "host" for chia and will fill you up nicely, with good nutrition as well.

Yield:	Prep time:	Cook time:	Serving size:
6 muffins	20 minutes	20 minutes	1 muffin
Each serving has:			
330 calories	120 calories from fat	14 g total fat	7 g saturated fat
100 mg cholesterol	440 mg sodium	39 g carbohydrates	6 g fiber
14 g sugar	14 g protein	185 mg potassium	203 mg calcium

1 cup buckwheat flour

$^1/_2$ cup cornmeal

$2^1/_2$ tsp. baking powder

$^1/_4$ tsp. sea salt

$1^1/_4$ cups 2% milk (or your favorite dairy substitute)

$^1/_2$ stick ($^1/_4$ cup) butter, melted

2 large eggs

4 TB. chia seeds

1 cup aged white cheddar cheese, shredded

$^1/_4$ cup honey

1 bunch chives, thinly sliced

1. Preheat the oven to 400°F. Lightly grease 6 muffin tins or line with paper cupcake liners.

2. In a large bowl, mix buckwheat flour, cornmeal, baking powder, and sea salt.

3. In a medium bowl, whisk together 2% milk, butter, eggs, and chia seeds.

4. Pour wet mixture into dry mixture and incorporate until combined. Fold in aged white cheddar cheese and sliced chives.

5. Divide batter evenly into muffin tins or cups.

6. Bake for 18 to 20 minutes or until toothpick comes out clean when inserted into the center of corn muffin.

7. Allow to cool on a cooling rack for about 5 minutes.

8. Garnish corn muffins with honey and chives and serve.

Maple-Blueberry-Chia Muffins

Nothing says breakfast like the great taste of maple and blueberries, plus the added nutrition of chia!

Yield:	Prep time:	Cook time:	Serving size:
12 muffins	8 minutes	30 minutes	1 muffin

Each serving has:			
120 calories	25 calories from fat	2.5 g total fat	1 g saturated fat
0 mg cholesterol	230 mg sodium	18 g carbohydrates	3 g fiber
2 g sugar	6 g protein	81 mg potassium	53 mg calcium

2 TB. ground flaxseeds

$^3/_4$ cup whole-wheat flour

$^3/_4$ cup plus 2 TB. all-purpose flour

$^1/_4$ cup vanilla protein powder

$1^1/_2$ tsp. baking powder

1 tsp. ground cinnamon

$^1/_2$ tsp. ground cloves

$^1/_2$ tsp. ground nutmeg

$^1/_2$ tsp. baking soda

$^1/_4$ tsp. sea salt

$^1/_4$ cup white beans

$^1/_2$ cup liquid egg substitute

$^1/_2$ cup sugar-free maple syrup

$^1/_2$ cup fat-free buttermilk

$^1/_2$ cup vanilla Greek yogurt

1 tsp. chia seeds

1 TB. Splenda

2 tsp. vegetable oil

2 tsp. orange zest

1 TB. orange juice

$1^1/_2$ cups fresh blueberries

1. Preheat the oven to 400°F. Coat 12 muffin cups with cooking spray.

2. In a large bowl, whisk flaxseeds, whole-wheat flour, all-purpose flour, vanilla protein powder, baking powder, cinnamon, cloves, nutmeg, baking soda, and sea salt until blended. Set aside.

3. In a food processor or blender, purée white beans.

4. In a medium bowl, whisk liquid egg substitute and sugar-free maple syrup until smooth. Add fat-free buttermilk, vanilla Greek yogurt, chia seeds, Splenda, vegetable oil, white bean purée, orange zest, and orange juice until blended.

5. Make a well in dry ingredients, add wet ingredients, and stir with a rubber spatula just until moistened.

6. Fold in blueberries and scoop batter into the prepared muffin cups.

7. Bake muffins until the tops are golden brown and spring back when touched lightly, about 15 to 25 minutes.

8. Let muffins cool in the pan for 5 minutes. Loosen edges and turn out onto a wire rack to cool slightly.

9. Serve.

 FOOD FOR THOUGHT

Flaxseeds are a good source of omega-3 fatty acids, so try using flaxseeds or flaxseed oil in your diet every day. Don't go crazy with it, but 1 teaspoon of flaxseed oil drizzled on your eggs in the morning or put in a smoothie or protein shake can help you on your quest to achieving a healthier you.

Apple-Cinnamon-Chia Muffins

Crisp apple and warm cinnamon come together in these muffins that are a pleasant reminder of autumn.

Yield:	Prep time:	Cook time:	Serving size:
12 muffins	10 minutes	20 minutes	1 muffin

Each serving has:			
90 calories	30 calories from fat	3.5 g total fat	1 g saturated fat
0 mg cholesterol	220 mg sodium	13 g carbohydrates	2 g fiber
3 g sugar	4 g protein	39 mg potassium	26 mg calcium

$^1/_4$ cup brown sugar Splenda

$^1/_4$ cup whole-wheat flour

Pinch ground cinnamon

2 TB. reduced-fat margarine

3 TB. rolled oats

2 TB. puréed white beans

$^1/_2$ cup Splenda

1 tsp. chia seeds

2 tsp. vanilla extract

$^1/_4$ cup liquid egg substitute

$^1/_2$ cup all-purpose flour

$^1/_4$ cup whole-wheat flour

2 TB. vanilla protein powder

$^1/_2$ tsp. baking powder

$^1/_2$ tsp. baking soda

$^1/_2$ tsp. sea salt

$^1/_4$ cup vanilla Greek yogurt

2 TB. fat-free buttermilk

2 medium apples, cut into $^1/_4$-in. chunks

1. Preheat the oven to 375°F. Line 12 muffin cups with paper or foil liners.

2. In a large bowl, beat on medium brown sugar Splenda, whole-wheat flour, and cinnamon with a mixer fitted with a paddle attachment.

3. Add reduced-fat margarine and beat on low until crumb mixture forms. Add rolled oats and work in with your hands. Put mixture into a small bowl, and set aside.

4. In a large bowl, beat on medium puréed white beans, Splenda, chia seeds, and vanilla extract until light and fluffy. Add liquid egg substitute and beat on medium to combine, scraping sides of bowl.

5. In a 4-cup measuring cup, whisk all-purpose flour, whole wheat flour, vanilla protein powder, baking powder, baking soda, and sea salt.

6. Add flour mixture, vanilla Greek yogurt, and fat-free buttermilk to white bean–chia mixture and beat on low speed just until blended, scraping down the sides of bowl after 5 seconds. Stir in apple chunks.

7. Spoon a slightly heaping ⅛ cup batter into each muffin cup and sprinkle topping mixture evenly over each.

8. Place in the oven and bake for about 20 minutes or until muffins are lightly browned and top springs back after being pushed.

9. Remove from muffin cups and serve warm.

Cherry-Pecan-Chia Scones

These scones taste like cherry pie, only better!

Yield:	Prep time:	Cook time:	Serving size:
16 scones	8 minutes	10 minutes	1 scone

Each serving has:			
140 calories	30 calories from fat	3.5 g total fat	0 g saturated fat
0 mg cholesterol	290 mg sodium	22 g carbohydrates	2 g fiber
4 g sugar	5 g protein	67 mg potassium	46 mg calcium

Pan spray	1/4 cup vanilla protein powder
1/4 cup liquid egg substitute	1/3 cup Splenda
1 cup reduced-fat buttermilk	1 tsp. chia seeds
2 TB. canola oil	1 TB. baking powder
2 tsp. grated orange zest	1 tsp. sea salt
1/2 cup rolled oats	1/2 cup dried cherries
1 1/4 cups whole-wheat flour	1/4 cup chopped pecans
1 1/2 cups all-purpose flour	

1. Preheat the oven to 350°F. Coat a cookie sheet with pan spray and set aside.

2. In a small bowl, beat liquid egg substitute and reduced-fat buttermilk.

3. Add canola oil and orange zest and mix to combine.

4. In a large bowl, combine rolled oats, whole-wheat flour, all-purpose flour, vanilla protein powder, Splenda, chia seeds, baking powder, and sea salt.

5. Stir buttermilk mixture into dry ingredients and mix just until dough comes together; don't overmix.

6. Fold in cherries and pecans.

7. Scoop heaping tablespoons of dough onto the prepared cookie sheet and bake for 10 minutes or until slightly golden on top.

8. Serve warm.

 FOOD FOR THOUGHT

Dried cherries are an anti-inflammatory, making them a good choice to add to dishes and eat as a healthy snack.

Crispy Chia-Maple Bacon

Bacon is famously savory and delicious and is often cited by vegans as their main reason for missing (or returning to) eating meat. Adding maple syrup to it adds sweetness and only makes it better. By also including chia, you have something with nutritional goodness and great flavor.

Yield:	Prep time:	Cook time:	Serving size:
12 pieces bacon	5 minutes	24 minutes	2 pieces bacon

Each serving has:			
250 calories	200 calories from fat	22 g total fat	7 g saturated fat
30 mg cholesterol	380 mg sodium	9 g carbohydrates	2 g fiber
7 g sugar	6 g protein	101 mg potassium	29 mg calcium

12 strips bacon	Freshly cracked black pepper
4 TB. maple syrup	2 TB. plus 1 tsp. chia seeds

1. On a baking sheet, arrange slices of bacon so they're not touching one another.

2. Turn the oven to 400°F and place the baking sheet in the oven.

3. Bake for 14 minutes or until almost done and remove briefly.

4. With a basting brush or other tool, brush maple syrup and black pepper on top of bacon. Sprinkle chia seeds on top.

5. Put baking sheet back in the oven and cook until bacon is crisp, about 10 minutes.

6. Remove immediately from the pan, as hot grease will otherwise continue to cook bacon, and serve.

Lunches

Getting your chia in early each day is crucial to help chia do its job of settling into your stomach. By keeping chia in your system, you reduce your appetite and smooth out the flow of energy into your body. If you don't exercise during the day, chia helps you moderate your food consumption to fit; if you do exercise, chia delivers steady energy.

I've found it easier to get in my first tablespoon of chia at breakfast than to get another quantity in at lunch. I'm often out and about, frequently with other people, so it's easy to leave my chia seeds at home or "forget" to add them to my meal when I'm sitting with other people.

The recipes in this chapter are a big part of the answer. You can easily prepare delicious food that's easy to eat, portable, and incorporates a healthy portion of chia.

These recipes are great for eating at home or preparing at home and traveling with you to work or elsewhere.

In This Chapter

- Bread and bagel sandwiches with chia
- Chia chili and pasta
- Soup and salads with chia for lunch

Chia-Jelly, Peanut Butter, and Banana Sandwich

Peanut butter and jelly is a famously easy-to-make and easy-to-carry sandwich. The rich nuttiness of peanut butter and the sweetness of jelly make it delicious as well. In this version, we add the sweetness and richness of banana and the nutritional goodness of chia seeds.

Yield:	Prep time:	Serving size:	
1 sandwich	5 minutes	1 sandwich	
Each serving has:			
550 calories	180 calories from fat	20 g total fat	3 g saturated fat
0 mg cholesterol	460 mg sodium	80 g carbohydrates	9 g fiber
33 g sugar	17 g protein	465 mg potassium	238 mg calcium

2 slices multi-grain bread

2 TB. peanut butter

1 tsp. chia seeds

1 TB. jelly or fresh fruit preserves

$^1/_2$ banana, peeled and sliced in half and lengthwise

1. Take multi-grain bread slices and spread peanut butter on one side of each.

2. In a small bowl, stir chia seeds and jelly. Spread chia-jelly on other half of bread slices.

3. Place banana on peanut butter half, put chia-jelly half on top, and serve.

 CHIA CAUTION

Peanut butter and jelly sandwiches are famous for sticking to the roof of your mouth. Every ingredient in them—peanut butter, jelly, and bread—is sticky in this way, and the combination is powerful. Each of these ingredients also needs water to digest. Add chia, which needs even more water to digest, and it becomes very important indeed to have lots of water. Try to have a couple of full, 8-ounce glasses with this sandwich.

The Big Chia-eese

Grilled cheese is delicious, bringing out the best of the bread you use with the rich, tangy flavor of cheese. Adding the smooth, tangy taste of tomatoes and the earthy richness of quince paste only ups the taste.

Yield:	Prep time:	Cook time:	Serving size:
1 sandwich	5 minutes	2 to 3 minutes	1 sandwich
Each serving has:			
650 calories	210 calories from fat	24 g total fat	14 g saturated fat
55 mg cholesterol	1,290 mg sodium	87 g carbohydrates	6 g fiber
15 g sugar	23 g protein	434 mg potassium	172 mg calcium

2 slices sourdough bread	1 tsp. chia seeds
1/4 cup goat cheese	1 TB. butter
3 slices ripe tomato	1/4 tsp. sea salt
2 tsp. quince paste	1/4 tsp. cracked black pepper

1. Take sourdough bread slices and spread 1/2 of goat cheese on one side of each.

2. Place sliced tomatoes on one bread slice and quince paste on the other bread slice. Sprinkle chia seeds evenly over tomatoes.

3. In a medium skillet on medium-low heat, melt butter. Place sandwich in pan and cook about 2 to 3 minutes on each side or until golden brown.

4. Move sandwich to a plate, season with sea salt and black pepper, and serve.

 SEEDS OF CHANGE

You'll really notice if you use good tomatoes in this recipe. Heirloom or homegrown tomatoes are among the kinds that are likely to have richer flavor, making a better sandwich.

Bagel with Chia-Chive Cream Cheese and Salmon

The doughy goodness of bagels seems a natural fit for the creamy smoothness and richness of cream cheese. Adding the delicious, meaty taste of salmon and the tangy bite of capers makes for a delicious small meal.

Yield:	Prep time:	Serving size:	
1 bagel	10 minutes	1 bagel	

Each serving has:			
550 calories	120 calories from fat	14 g total fat	4 g saturated fat
95 mg cholesterol	720 mg sodium	59 g carbohydrates	5 g fiber
9 g sugar	48 g protein	709 mg potassium	184 mg calcium

1 TB. fresh, thinly sliced chives

$1/2$ tsp. lemon zest, grated

1 tsp. lemon juice

1 tsp. capers

1 tsp. chia seeds

1 TB. cream cheese

1 bagel (your choice), sliced in half

2 oz. smoked salmon slices

3 round slices cucumber

2 ($1/4$-in.) slices tomato

1 thin slice red onion

1. In a small bowl, mix chives, lemon zest, lemon juice, capers, chia seeds, and cream cheese.

2. Spread both bagel halves with mixture. Place, in order, sliced salmon slices, cucumber, tomato, and red onion on top of one half of the bagel. Place other half of bagel on top.

3. Slice in half and serve.

Sautéed Portobello and Tempeh Sandwich with Thai Chia-Chili Sauce

Portobello makes a great replacement for meat in many dishes, such as this sandwich. Its rich, earthy, and meaty flavor and texture can help you "go veg" for a meal, for a day, or maybe for years to come.

Yield:	Prep time:	Cook time:	Serving size:
1 sandwich	10 minutes	10 minutes	1 sandwich

Each serving has:			
690 calories	450 calories from fat	51 g total fat	7 g saturated fat
0 mg cholesterol	620 mg sodium	59 g carbohydrates	3 g fiber
20 g sugar	17 g protein	544 mg potassium	105 mg calcium

2 TB. extra-virgin olive oil

1 medium to large portobello mushroom

1 (2-oz.) slice organic tempeh

$1/4$ tsp. sea salt

$1/4$ tsp. cracked black pepper

1 large slice romaine lettuce, washed and patted dry on a clean cloth

1 (4-in.) square focaccia bread, sliced in half

1 TB. sesame oil

2 TB. Thai chili sauce

1 tsp. chia seeds

1. Heat up a medium skillet over medium heat. Add extra-virgin olive oil.

2. Add portobello mushroom and tempeh and sauté for 5 minutes on one side, seasoning with sea salt and black pepper.

3. Flip them over and cook for another 5 minutes. Remove from the skillet and set aside.

4. Place romaine lettuce slice and on bottom half of focaccia bread.

5. Drizzle cooked tempeh and portobello mushroom with sesame oil and place on top of romaine lettuce.

6. Stir chia seeds into Thai chili sauce and drizzle over top of sandwich. Cover with other focaccia bread half and serve.

Beef, Cheese, and Cucumber Sandwich with Chia

The rich flavor of beef and the zestiness of cheese combine with the cool crunch of cucumber to make for a satisfying sandwich. Using pita pockets helps you keep the serving size reasonable.

Yield:	**Prep time:**	**Serving size:**	
4 sandwiches	10 minutes	1 sandwich	
Each serving has:			
330 calories	70 calories from fat	8 g total fat	2.5 g saturated fat
40 mg cholesterol	760 mg sodium	42 g carbohydrates	6 g fiber
4 g sugar	22 g protein	252 mg potassium	180 mg calcium

4 (6^1/$_2$-in.) rounds pita bread

1 large tomato

1 medium cucumber

4 leaves lettuce

^{1}/$_2$ lb. sliced beef

4 TB. bleu cheese

4 TB. chia seeds

1. Cut top ^{1}/$_2$ inch off pita rounds to open them.

2. Slice tomato into 8 slices.

3. Slice cucumber into 16 slices.

4. In each pita round, place 1 lettuce leaf, 2 slices tomato, 4 slices cucumber, ¼ of sliced beef, 1 tablespoon of bleu cheese, and 1 tablespoon chia seeds.

5. Put on plates and serve.

 CHIA CAUTION

If you're going to save some of the sandwiches for later, don't add the tomato until just before eating, or the tomato juice can soak through the pita and make a mess.

Chia Pasta E Fagioli

Pasta is delicious and filling, but pasta dishes can suffer from a lack of nutritional oomph. This dish uses the bite of onion, the crunchiness of carrots and celeries, the rich flavor of chicken stock, and the tangy goodness of tomatoes to make a nutritionally rich and tasty dish.

Yield:	Prep time:	Cook time:	Serving size:
4 bowls pasta	40 minutes	45 minutes	1 bowl pasta

Each serving has:			
510 calories	190 calories from fat	121 g total fat	4.5 g saturated fat
15 mg cholesterol	870 mg sodium	60 g carbohydrates	8 g fiber
14 g sugar	20 g protein	1,028 mg potassium	194 mg calcium

$^1/_4$ cup extra-virgin olive oil

1 small onion, finely chopped

1 carrot, finely chopped

1 stalk celery, finely chopped

4 cloves garlic, minced

1 qt. chicken or vegetable stock

$^1/_2$ cup cannellini beans

5 tomatoes, peeled, seeded, and diced small

1 cup ditalini pasta

1 cup chopped Italian flat-leaf parsley

4 tsp. chia seeds

1 tsp. sea salt

1 tsp. cracked black pepper

$^1/_4$ tsp. crushed red chili flakes

2 TB. grated Parmesan cheese

1. In heavy, medium saucepot over medium-low heat, heat extra-virgin olive oil.

2. Add onion, carrot, and celery and cook until soft and translucent. Add garlic and stir for 2 minutes.

3. Add chicken broth, cannellini beans, and tomatoes and simmer for about 20 minutes.

4. Add ditalini pasta and cook until al dente, about 8 to 9 minutes. Turn off the heat.

5. Add Italian flat-leaf parsley and chia seeds and season with sea salt and black pepper.

6. Garnish pasta with a drizzle of extra-virgin olive oil, red chili flakes, and shaved Parmesan cheese and serve.

Slow-Cooked Chia Beef Chili

Chili combines the rich bulk of beans and the satisfying, chewy richness of beef to make for a delicious dish. It's one of the very best dishes for stretching a small amount of meat into a big, satisfying serving.

Yield:	Prep time:	Cook time:	Serving size:
2 bowls chili	30 minutes	7 to 8 hours	1 bowl chili

Each serving has:			
410 calories	120 calories from fat	14 g total fat	4.5 g saturated fat
70 mg cholesterol	450 mg sodium	30 g carbohydrates	8 g fiber
13 g sugar	28 g protein	1,001 mg potassium	134 mg calcium

$^3/_4$ cup red wine	2 carrots, diced medium
2 cups beef broth	8 cloves garlic, chopped
4 plum tomatoes chopped, diced medium	3 sprigs fresh thyme
	1 sprig rosemary
1 lb. beef stew meat	2 bay leaves
1 large onion, diced medium	4 tsp. chia seeds
1 shallot, minced	$^1/_2$ tsp. sea salt
3 stalks celery, diced medium	$^1/_2$ tsp. cracked black pepper

1. In a large slow cooker, place red wine, beef broth, and plum tomatoes. Set heat to low.

2. Add beef stew meat, onion, shallot, celery, carrots, garlic, thyme, rosemary, bay leaves, and chia seeds and cook on low for 7 to 8 hours or until tender.

3. Remove bay leaves, thyme, and rosemary, sprinkle with sea salt and black pepper, and serve.

Chia French Onion Soup

French onion soup combines the zestiness of onions with the rich flavor of Calvados and the earthy, tangy flavor of gruyère cheese. Adding chia provides nutrition without changing the texture or flavor much at all.

Yield:	Prep time:	Cook time:	Serving size:
4 bowls soup	15 minutes	2 hours	1 bowl soup

Each serving has:			
440 calories	210 calories from fat	24 g total fat	14 g saturated fat
65 mg cholesterol	760 mg sodium	33 g carbohydrates	6 g fiber
11 g sugar	19 g protein	811 mg potassium	430 mg calcium

½ stick (¼ cup) unsalted butter	¼ tsp. sea salt
2 lb. yellow onion, sliced in half rings	¼ tsp. cracked black pepper
¼ cup Calvados or applejack brandy	8 tsp. chia seeds
4 cups veal, beef, or chicken stock	4 slices sourdough French bread
2 sprigs thyme	½ cup grated gruyère cheese
2 bay leaves	4 tsp. Parmesan cheese

1. In a medium saucepot on low heat, add butter and yellow onion and caramelize for 1 hour and 30 minutes, making sure to stir often with wooden spoon.

2. Deglaze onions with Calvados. Add veal stock, thyme, and bay leaves and cook for 30 minutes.

3. Add sea salt and black pepper. Pour soup into bowls or mugs and add 2 teaspoons chia seeds to each serving.

4. Place 1 slice sourdough French bread, ¼ of gruyere cheese, and 1 teaspoon Parmesan cheese on top of each bowl.

5. Set an oven to broil. Place the bowls on a cookie sheet and slide into the oven. Broil until cheese is bubbling, melted, and golden brown. Remove the cookie sheet carefully and handle the bowls carefully, as they will be hot. Serve.

 SEEDS OF CHANGE

French onion soup is famously tricky to eat because the melted cheese is so stringy. Consider putting out cloth napkins and setting an example for people eating with you by tucking one into your collar, underneath your chin.

Bean and Chia-Cheddar Taco Salad

Taco salad combines the rich flavor of beans; the cool flavor of lettuce; the tanginess of tomato; the smooth, satisfying flavor of sour cream; and more into a tasty and filling vegetarian dish.

Yield:	Prep time:	Cook time:	Serving size:
2 bowls taco salad	25 minutes	15 minutes	1 bowl taco salad

Each serving has:			
410 calories	130 calories from fat	14 g total fat	3 g saturated fat
10 mg cholesterol	740 mg sodium	54 g carbohydrates	11 g fiber
7 g sugar	19 g protein	211 mg potassium	207 mg calcium

1 (16-oz.) can chili beans	1 medium tomato, diced small
4 tsp. chia seeds	1/2 cup chopped scallions
3/4 cup salsa Fresca	1/4 cup black olives, sliced
3/4 cup corn chips	2 TB. chopped cilantro
1 cup shredded cheddar cheese	1/4 cup shredded carrots
2 cups romaine lettuce, washed, drained, and torn into bite-size pieces	1/4 cup sour cream

1. Preheat the oven to 350°F.

2. In a small saucepot, place chili beans and cook over low to medium heat until hot.

3. In a small bowl, add chia seeds and salsa Fresca and stir. Set aside.

4. On a plate, arrange corn chips. Spoon chili beans on top of chips. Add shredded cheese.

5. Place plate in the oven and bake until cheese is melted.

6. Top with romaine lettuce, tomato, scallions, black olives, cilantro, shredded carrots, and sour cream and serve immediately.

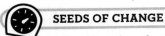 **SEEDS OF CHANGE**

To reduce the calorie count of this dish, consider replacing the sour cream with Greek yogurt.

Butter Lettuce Salad with Paté and Chia-Mustard Vinaigrette

This salad is hearty and delicious, with the paté adding savor without a lot of meat per serving.

Yield:	Prep time:	Serving size:	
2 bowls salad	15 minutes	1 bowl salad	

Each serving has:			
350 calories	260 calories from fat	29 g total fat	4.5 g saturated fat
160 mg cholesterol	550 mg sodium	17 g carbohydrates	1 g fiber
9 g sugar	5 g protein	51 mg potassium	19 mg calcium

1 head butter lettuce, washed, dried, and leaves separated	6 TB. extra-virgin olive oil
1 egg yolk	1/4 tsp. sea salt
1 TB. grainy Dijon mustard	1/4 tsp. cracked black pepper
2 tsp. chia seeds	14 cornichons
1 1/2 tsp. minced shallots	14 dry-cured black olives, pitted
2 TB. champagne vinegar	2 (2-oz.) slices prepared chicken liver paté

1. In a large bowl, place butter lettuce.

2. In a blender, add egg yolk, grainy Dijon mustard, chia seeds, shallots, and champagne vinegar and blend on emulsify setting, drizzling in extra-virgin olive oil to form an emulsion. Season with sea salt and black pepper.

3. Add dressing to bowl of lettuce and toss to coat. Arrange salad on two plates and garnish with cornichons and black olives. Place one slice chicken liver paté on each plate and serve.

 FOOD FOR THOUGHT

It's a good idea to add chia to salad dressing, as it reduces the caloric impact of each spoonful. At the same time, if you're gradually reducing the amount of salad dressing you use, consider sprinkling 1 teaspoon of chia seeds over your salad. If you add it to your salad, be sure to drink one full glass of water along with your meal to help you feel full sooner and to meet the need for water to help digest the chia seeds.

Soups

A cup of soup gets a different texture if you add 1 tablespoon of chia seeds to it; the effect isn't dramatic, but it is noticeable. It's the kind of thing you might see doing for a dish you're eating alone, but less so if you're sharing the dish with others who aren't chia savvy.

In a bowl of chili, which already has several different textures in it, the same effect is less noticeable. You can add a bit of additional water to keep the overall consistency the same and serve the dish to people without worrying about whether they'll notice the difference.

Try going with the chia recommendations in the recipes, but also feel free to experiment after you've made it once or twice to see what works best for you and others you're eating with.

In This Chapter

- Chia broth and stock you can use as a base
- Healthy chia vegetable soups
- Hearty beef stew with chia

Quick Chia Seed Chicken Broth

Chicken broth is the basis for a very wide range of recipes. It has a rich and fatty flavor without actually containing all that much fat. This recipe uses store-bought chicken broth and a store-bought roast chicken plus chia to achieve delicious results at a low cost and in less than an hour.

Yield:	Prep time:	Cook time:	Serving size:
3$\frac{1}{2}$ quarts chicken broth	20 minutes	40 minutes	1 cup chicken broth

Each serving has:			
130 calories	80 calories from fat	9 g total fat	2 g saturated fat
45 mg cholesterol	690 mg sodium	5 g carbohydrates	2 g fiber
2 g sugar	10 g protein	71 mg potassium	31 mg calcium

2 qt. store-bought chicken broth

1 qt. water

5 TB. chia seeds or 2 cups chia gel

1 store-bought roast chicken

3 tsp. vegetable oil

2 large onions, cut into a medium dice

2 large carrots, peeled and cut into rounds or half rounds

2 large stalks celery, sliced $\frac{1}{4}$ in. thick

1 tsp. dried thyme leaves

1. In a large pot with a lid, combine chicken broth, water, and chia seeds and bring to a simmer over medium heat.

2. While heating broth and water, remove chicken meat from roast chicken and set aside.

3. Put skin and bones in the pot, cover, and simmer on medium for 20 minutes.

4. Strain broth through a colander or cheesecloth back into the pot. Discard skin and bones.

5. Add vegetable oil, onions, carrots, and celery and sauté on medium-high heat until vegetables soften, about 8 to 10 minutes.

6. Add chicken meat and thyme and return to a simmer.

7. Refrigerate and use within 1 week.

FOOD FOR THOUGHT

There's an old saying that you shouldn't count your chickens before they're hatched. Perhaps you also shouldn't count your chickens before you know how they're raised. Consider "sourcing" your chickens from providers who commit to not raising chickens in cramped and unsanitary conditions. The label you might look for here is "free range," but research the specific provider to find out what that means before putting too much stock in it (no pun intended).

Quick Chia Seed Beef Stock

Beef stock is very widely used, but not quite as much as chicken broth (see previous recipe). Still, beef stock is a very effective way to get the goodness of beef without overconsuming it. Beef stock adds a rich, hearty, savory flavor to dishes, even those that have no other meat in them of any kind. You can also eat it directly as a soup with some vegetables.

Yield:	Prep time:	Cook time:	Serving size:
8 cups beef stock	20 minutes	6 hours	$^1/_2$ cup beef stock

Each serving has:			
190 calories	100 calories from fat	11 g total fat	4 g saturated fat
35 mg cholesterol	500 mg sodium	8 g carbohydrates	3 g fiber
2 g sugar	15 g protein	351 mg potassium	43 mg calcium

1 large onion	8 whole black peppercorns
3 large carrots	1 large tomato
1 medium potato	1 bay leaf
6 lb. beef soup bones	1 TB. sea salt
2 stalks celery, including some leaves	2 tsp. dried thyme
$^1/_3$ cup chia seeds	2 cloves garlic
4 sprigs fresh parsley	3 qt. water
$^1/_2$ cup chopped parsnips	

1. Preheat the oven to 350°F.

2. Remove end from onion and tops from carrots. Quarter onion and cut carrots into 1-inch chunks.

3. Place beef soup bones, carrots, and onions on a baking sheet and bake in the oven for about 30 minutes, until bones are well browned. Drain fat away.

4. Scrub potato and cut into 1-inch chunks, chop celery stalks into 1-inch lengths, and place in a large pot.

5. Add chia seeds, parsley, parsnips, black peppercorns, tomato, bay leaf, sea salt, thyme, garlic, beef soup bones, carrots, onions, and water.

6. Bring mixture to a boil over medium-high heat and then simmer over low heat for 5 hours.

7. Strain beef stock through a cheesecloth. Discard meat and bones, vegetable pieces, and seasoning pieces.

8. Refrigerate and use within 2 weeks.

Quick Noodle and Vegetable Chia Soup

Noodles provide a satisfying base for the tangy, zesty, and sweet flavors of the bell pepper, olives, and corn in this soup.

Yield:	Prep time:	Cook time:	Serving size:
6 bowls soup	10 minutes	10 minutes	1 bowl soup

Each serving has:			
210 calories	5 calories from fat	0.5 g total fat	0 g saturated fat
0 mg cholesterol	700 mg sodium	44 g carbohydrates	3 g fiber
9 g sugar	7 g protein	178 mg potassium	21 mg calcium

1 green bell pepper	1 cup black olives
1 medium onion	$^1/_2$ cup peas
1 cup mushrooms	6 cups vegetable broth
1 clove garlic	$^1/_2$ tsp. sea salt
6 cups water	$^1/_2$ tsp. ground pepper
1 cup corn	$^1/_2$ lb. vermicelli pasta

1. Cut green bell pepper, onion, and mushrooms into small pieces.

2. Mash garlic into a paste.

3. In a large pot over high heat, pour in water and bring to a boil.

4. Reduce heat to medium. Add green bell pepper, onion, mushrooms, corn, black olives, peas, vegetable broth, sea salt, and black pepper and cook for 10 minutes, stirring occasionally.

5. Add vermicelli pasta and cook until noodles soften, about 10 minutes.

6. Spoon into bowls and serve.

 SEEDS OF CHANGE

This soup is very flexible. You can use all different kinds of noodles and in-season vegetables and then garnish with Greek yogurt or avocado slices. You can even brown $^1/_2$ pound of beef or a few slices of bacon and add it to the soup.

Spicy Tortilla Vegetable Soup with Chia-Lime Sour Cream

The cool sour cream offsets the spiciness of this fun and nutritious dish. For a lower-calorie alternative, you can use plain yogurt or Greek yogurt in place of the sour cream.

Yield:	Prep time:	Cook time:	Serving size:
4 bowls soup and 1 cup sour cream	20 minutes	35 minutes	1 bowl soup and $^1/_4$ cup sour cream

Each serving has:			
440 calories	240 calories from fat	27 g total fat	9 g saturated fat
40 mg cholesterol	370 mg sodium	41 g carbohydrates	9 g fiber
15 g sugar	8 g protein	849 mg potassium	153 mg calcium

3 red bell peppers

4 large ripe tomatoes

8 tomatillos, peel removed

1 jalapeño

$^1/_4$ cup extra-virgin olive oil

$^1/_2$ cup chopped onions

7 cloves garlic, peeled

2 TB. ancho chili powder

2 cups vegetable or chicken broth

4 corn tortillas

$^1/_4$ cup chopped cilantro

Sea salt

Ground black pepper

4 tsp. chia seeds

1 cup sour cream

$^1/_4$ cup fresh-squeezed lime juice

$^1/_4$ cup chopped cilantro

2 limes, fresh squeezed and quartered

1. On a grill or cast-iron skillet, dry roast red bell peppers, tomatoes, tomatillos, and jalapeño until charred. Set aside to cool off, about 5 minutes.

2. Peel and de-seed red bell peppers and jalapeño.

3. In a medium sauce pot or soup pot over medium heat, add extra-virgin olive oil, onions, garlic, roasted red bell peppers, roasted tomatoes, roasted tomatillos and roasted jalapeño, stirring occasionally. Season with salt and pepper to taste and add ancho chili powder.

4. Add vegetable broth, cover, and simmer for 30 minutes over low heat or until soft.

5. While soup is simmering, in a sauté pan, add some oil and brown corn tortillas on both sides.

6. Carefully pour soup base into a blender. Add browned tortillas and purée until smooth. (If you like the soup base thinner, add some more broth; if you like it thicker, simply purée more tortilla until you reach the desired consistency.) Set aside.

7. In a medium bowl, whisk together chia seeds, sour cream, and lime juice. Wait 10 minutes to allow the flavors to combine.

8. Pour soup into bowls, add sour cream to top, garnish with cilantro and lime quarters, and serve.

Napolitano Minestrone Soup with Chia

This soup has a wide range of hearty vegetables you can vary based on what's available seasonally. You can also eat this filling soup hot or cold.

Yield:	Prep time:	Cook time:	Serving size:
6 bowls soup	20 minutes	50 minutes	1 bowl soup

Each serving has:			
320 calories	120 calories from fat	13 g total fat	2.5 g saturated fat
5 mg cholesterol	400 mg sodium	43 g carbohydrates	9 g fiber
9 g sugar	9 g protein	555 mg potassium	184 mg calcium

1 lb. butternut squash	6 medium fresh ripe tomatoes, diced
1 cup canned, drained, and rinsed cannellini beans	2 cups vegetable broth
$^1/_2$ cup green peas, shelled	Sea salt
1 small rutabaga, diced	Ground black pepper
1 small turnip, diced	$^1/_2$ cup short-grain white rice
1 small carrot, diced	4 TB. chia seeds
2 small stalks celery, diced	$^1/_2$ cup chopped Italian flat-leaf parsley
1 medium onion, diced small	$^1/_4$ cup torn basil leaves
8 cloves garlic, chopped	4 TB. Parmesan cheese
$^1/_4$ cup extra-virgin olive oil	

1. Remove rind and seeds from butternut squash and cut into cubes.

2. In a medium bowl, place butternut squash cubes, cannellini beans, green peas, rutabaga, turnip, carrot, and celery. Set aside.

3. In a medium sauté pan on medium heat, sauté onion and garlic in extra-virgin olive oil until translucent.

4. Add vegetables and stir occasionally for 10 minutes.

5. Add tomatoes and vegetable broth, season with sea salt and black pepper to taste, and simmer on medium for 20 minutes.

6. Add short-grain white rice and chia seeds and simmer for 20 more minutes, adding more sea salt and black pepper as necessary.

7. Pour into bowls and serve sprinkled with Italian flat-leaf parsley, basil, and Parmesan cheese.

Chia Zucchini and Toasted Garlic Purée Soup with Parmesan

This delicious and hearty soup gets you plenty of healthy elements and has a bit of that "stick to your ribs" quality that's rare in vegetarian dishes.

Yield:	Prep time:	Cook time:	Serving size:
6 bowls soup	20 minutes	20 minutes	1 bowl soup

Each serving has:			
220 calories	160 calories from fat	18 g total fat	3 g saturated fat
5 mg cholesterol	390 mg sodium	12 g carbohydrates	3 g fiber
4 g sugar	5 g protein	270 mg potassium	126 mg calcium

1 shallot, peeled and sliced	4 TB. chia seeds
6 to 8 cloves garlic, chopped	4 TB. Parmesan cheese to grate over finished soup
$^1/_4$ cup plus 2 TB. extra-virgin olive oil	Sea salt
4 cups zucchini, chopped and seeded	Ground black pepper
3 cups vegetable or chicken broth	$^1/_2$ cup chopped Italian flat-leaf parsley

1. In a medium saucepan over medium heat, sauté shallot and garlic in ¼ cup extra-virgin olive oil until golden brown.

2. Add zucchini and sauté until almost tender, about 5 minutes.

3. Add vegetable broth and bring to simmer. Simmer on medium until zucchini is fully tender, about 5 to 10 minutes.

4. In a blender, pour soup and blend on the purée setting while drizzling remaining 2 tablespoons extra-virgin olive oil.

5. Add chia seeds to puréed soup, and let settle for 10 minutes.

6. Pour into bowls, grate Parmesan cheese on top, add sea salt and black pepper to taste, garnish with Italian flat-leaf parsley, and serve.

 SEEDS OF CHANGE

Vegetarians include dairy products in their diets; vegans don't. For this delicious soup, leave off the Parmesan cheese to take this dish from vegetarian to vegan.

Ham and Bean Chia Soup

Combining meaty and flavorful ham with rich beans makes for a hearty meal where a small amount of meat goes a long way.

Yield:	Prep time:	Cook time:	Serving size:
6 bowls soup	5 minutes	25 minutes	1 bowl soup

Each serving has:			
320 calories	140 calories from fat	16 g total fat	6 g saturated fat
50 mg cholesterol	1,270 mg sodium	27 g carbohydrates	8 g fiber
6 g sugar	25 g protein	805 mg potassium	152 mg calcium

2 TB. olive oil	1 bay leaf
2 cups ham, diced	4 cups kale, sliced thin
1 medium onion, chopped	2 TB. chia seeds
2 garlic cloves, chopped fine	1/4 tsp. sea salt
2 tsp. fresh thyme leaves	1/4 tsp. black pepper
4 cups chicken broth	1 cup Greek yogurt
2 (15-oz.) cans white beans	

1. In a medium pot, mix olive oil, ham, onion, garlic, and thyme. Cook over medium heat until onion is softened, about 5 minutes.

2. Add chicken broth, white beans, bay leaf, kale, chia seeds, sea salt, and black pepper and cook for 20 minutes, stirring occasionally.

3. Pour into bowls, garnish with Greek yogurt, and serve.

 SEEDS OF CHANGE

If you don't care for ham, substitute the same amount of chicken or turkey, or about half as much beef, to get a similar feeling of meatiness along with a similar amount of fat, calories, and nutrition.

Pork and Green Pepper Stew with Chia

Pork and green peppers have a fairly subtle flavor, so the tanginess and heat of the jalapeño livens it up nicely.

Yield:	Prep time:	Cook time:	Serving size:
6 bowls soup	10 minutes	1 hour and 10 minutes	1 bowl soup

Each serving has:			
520 calories	250 calories from fat	28 g total fat	9 g saturated fat
145 mg cholesterol	1,130 mg sodium	15 g carbohydrates	2 g fiber
6 g sugar	46 g protein	737 mg potassium	31 mg calcium

2 TB. olive oil	1 green bell pepper, diced
2 lb. boneless pork shoulder cut into 1¹/₂-in. cubes	1 (16-oz.) can corn
2 cups chopped onions	1 TB. minced jalapeño
1 tsp. sea salt	2 cloves garlic, minced
1 tsp. ground cumin	1 TB. chia seeds
1 cup chicken broth	1 (16-oz.) jar salsa
	¹/₄ cup chopped fresh cilantro

1. Preheat the oven to 350°F.

2. In a medium frying pan over medium-high heat, heat olive oil.

3. Add pork, onions, sea salt, and cumin and cook until pork is browned on all sides, about 7 minutes.

4. Put browned pork in an oven-safe bowl.

5. Add chicken broth, green bell pepper, onions, corn, jalapeño, garlic, salsa, and cilantro. Cover and bake until pork is tender, about 1 hour.

6. Skim off any fat from the top and serve.

 SEEDS OF CHANGE

Any time you see green bell pepper in a sidebar, you can substitute red, yellow, or orange bell peppers. You can even use a combination to add some visual appeal. None of them are spicy, but the other colors all have more flavor than the green pepper. Each color of pepper has slightly different nutritional profile, so mixing up the colors also gives you more complete nutrition.

Chilled Cucumber Soup with Chia

Chilled soups yield up their flavors as you eat them. This cool, refreshing soup gets its creaminess from Greek yogurt instead of something with more fat and calories, such as, well, cream.

Yield:	Prep time:	Serving size:
4 bowls soup	1 hour and 15 minutes	1 bowl soup

Each serving has:			
180 calories	100 calories from fat	12 g total fat	9 g saturated fat
20 mg cholesterol	1,050 mg sodium	10 g carbohydrates	2 g fiber
8 g sugar	9 g protein	0 mg potassium	130 mg calcium

2 cucumbers	1 cup vegetable broth
4 green onions	2 TB. chia seeds
2 TB. dill	1 TB. sea salt
2 TB. parsley	1/2 lemon
2 cups Greek yogurt	

1. Dice cucumbers and slice green onions.

2. In a food processor, purée half of cucumber pieces, half of green onion slices, dill, and parsley.

3. In a large bowl, place purée mixture, remaining half of cucumber pieces, remaining half of green onion slices, Greek yogurt, vegetable broth, chia seeds, and sea salt and whisk to combine.

4. Squeeze lemon onto mixture and place in the refrigerator for 1 hour.

5. Pour into bowls and serve.

 SEEDS OF CHANGE

Make a full meal out of this soup by serving it with sandwiches, such as the Chia-Jelly, Peanut Butter, and Banana Sandwich (see Chapter 15).

CHAPTER 17

Lighter Fare

Getting 2 or 3 tablespoons of chia a day into your diet requires a multi-front strategy. Lighter fare, such as salads and snacks, are "side doors" for adding chia painlessly.

Adding 1 teaspoon of chia to just about any of these dishes is totally painless. That small amount of chia doesn't soak up much water (about 3 ounces of water for each teaspoon of chia), but over the course of the day, it adds up; each teaspoon you get is a big step toward your goal.

Adding a tablespoon of chia has more impact; a tablespoon of chia absorbs a little more than $1/2$ cup of water before you fully digest it. For these dishes, which don't have much fluid in them, the chia will absorb water from your body. This can make you feel quite thirsty, so have a glass of water on hand when consuming them.

As these recipes show, you'll get a feel over time for how much chia you can add to different dishes without affecting them much, depending on whether you're cooking for yourself, for friends, or for company that might not want to notice anything different at all about a dish.

In This Chapter

- Fresh salads with chia sauces and dressings
- Chia chips and crisps
- Chia snacks that satisfy your sweet tooth

Heirloom Tomato and Mozzarella Salad with Walnut-Chia-Basil Pesto

This refreshing salad incorporates a full tablespoon of chia per serving. Use the best tomatoes you can, as their tangy flavor is highlighted in this dish, along with the rich flavor of cheese and the delicious bite of pesto. You can use the pesto with other salads or on pizza or sandwiches.

Yield:	Prep time:	Serving size:	
6 bowls salad plus 2 TB. pesto	20 minutes	1 bowl salad plus 1 tsp. pesto	

Each serving has:			
280 calories	210 calories from fat	24 g total fat	8 g saturated fat
35 mg cholesterol	65 mg sodium	35 g carbohydrates	4 g fiber
2 g sugar	10 g protein	205 mg potassium	94 mg calcium

4 TB. chia seeds

4 TB. walnuts, toasted

3 cups fresh-picked basil, stems removed

6 cloves garlic, peeled

1/3 cup lemon juice

1 TB. lemon zest

2 TB. grated Pecorino Romano cheese

Sea salt

Cracked black pepper

1/4 cup extra-virgin olive oil

3/4 lb. fresh, ripe heirloom tomatoes, sliced in small wedges

1 1/4 cups (10 oz.) fresh mozzarella, *bocconcini*

1. In a blender, place chia seeds, walnuts, basil, garlic, lemon juice, lemon zest, Pecorino Romano cheese, sea salt to taste, and black pepper to taste and blend on purée setting.

2. Drizzle extra-virgin olive oil in a steady stream into the blender until everything is incorporated and emulsified.

3. Arrange tomato wedges and mozzarella on a platter, drizzle or spoon pesto over top, and serve.

 DEFINITION

Bocconcini means "small mouthfuls" in Italian. Bocconcini are little balls of mozzarella cheese. Back in the day, they were made exclusively from the milk of water buffalo. Today, cow's milk is in the mix. Like other mozzarellas, bocconcini have a mild flavor of their own and tend to absorb strong flavors from dishes they're included in. Bocconcini also tend to come packaged in whey or water, which is useful for combining with water-hungry chia seeds.

Tomato and Avocado Salad with Chia

A tangy but creamy tomato and avocado salad with chia combines all sorts of good things in one. Eat this as is, or add the same ingredients to lettuce and other greens—perhaps even a bit of meat, like solid albacore tuna—for a salad that will eat like a meal.

Yield:	Prep time:	Serving size:	
2 cups salad	10 minutes	$^1/_2$ cup salad	
Each serving has:			
120 calories	70 calories from fat	8 g total fat	1 g saturated fat
0 mg cholesterol	160 mg sodium	12 g carbohydrates	6 g fiber
5 g sugar	3 g protein	677 mg potassium	34 mg calcium

4 large tomatoes	$^1/_4$ tsp. sea salt
1 large avocado	$^1/_4$ tsp. cracked black pepper
2 tsp. chia seeds	

1. Remove end from tomatoes and dice.

2. Remove end from avocado, cut in half, remove pit, and dice insides.

3. In a medium bowl, combine diced tomatoes and avocado.

4. Add chia seeds, sea salt, and black pepper.

5. Divide into bowls and serve.

 FOOD FOR THOUGHT

Avocados are fattier than any fruit or vegetable around. Should you eschew them? A half cup of avocado is about one sixth of the fat and one twelfth the saturated fat recommended for an adult in their daily food intake. At the same time, it's a rich source of potassium, dietary fiber, and vitamin C.

Avocado punches above its weight when it comes to being fulfilling and nutritious, so don't be afraid to have avocados in your diet. You can even use avocado to serve as a much healthier substitute for part of the meat in your diet.

Chia Greek Salad with Tuna and Honey-Lemon Vinaigrette

The green salad, tuna salad, and dressing go great together and can be mixed and matched with other salads and dressings. The salad combines the sweet flavor of honey, the sharp flavor of shallots, and the bite of lemon juice, along with the savory flavor and texture of tuna. The tuna salad, which includes the chia seeds, can also be used for sandwiches.

Yield:	Prep time:	Serving size:	
6 bowls salad	20 minutes	1 bowl salad	
Each serving has:			
470 calories	330 calories from fat	37 g total fat	8 g saturated fat
30 mg cholesterol	290 mg sodium	26 g carbohydrates	6 g fiber
14 g sugar	12 g protein	505 mg potassium	201 mg calcium

1/4 cup fresh-squeezed lemon juice

Zest of 1 lemon

3 TB. honey

1 small shallot

Sea salt

Ground black pepper

3/4 cup extra-virgin olive oil

1 (5-oz.) can tuna in spring water

3 TB. chia seeds

1/4 cup celery, diced small

1/3 cup fresh oregano, chopped

2 tsp. garlic powder

3 TB. mayonnaise

1 head romaine lettuce

1 medium cucumber, sliced in half moons

1 medium red onion, sliced in thin rounds

1 large ripe tomato, diced medium

1 red bell pepper, diced medium

1/2 cup feta cheese

1. In a blender, place lemon juice, lemon zest, honey, shallot, sea salt to taste, and black pepper to taste and blend at medium speed, drizzling extra-virgin olive oil in slowly to form an emulsion. Season more as desired with sea salt and black pepper. Set aside.

2. Open can of tuna and place it and spring water into a medium bowl.

3. Flake tuna, add chia seeds, celery, oregano, garlic powder, and mayonnaise, and mix. Season more as desired with sea salt and black pepper. Set aside.

4. Tear, wash, and spin dry romaine lettuce. Place in a large bowl and add cucumber, red onion, tomato, and red bell pepper.

5. Place salad on plates, add one scoop of tuna salad to each, crumble feta cheese on top, and serve.

 FOOD FOR THOUGHT

Omega-3 fatty acids are desirable dietary building blocks for heart health. Modern practices, such as raising cattle in feed lots, increases the proportion of omega-6 fatty acids and decreases omega-3s, throwing the proportion out of whack. Therefore, you should try to augment your diet with omega-3-rich foods, such as chia, tuna fish, salmon, and mackerel. You want wild fish—salmon, for instance—not farmed, because the wild ones have more omega-3s. Among the different types of tuna you can buy, solid albacore tuna has more omega-3s than other kinds of tuna.

Chia Green Salad

With this salad, you get the wholesome crunchiness of romaine lettuce and the clean, fresh taste of cucumbers and green peppers.

Yield:	Prep time:	Serving size:	
3 cups salad	10 minutes	1 cup salad	
Each serving has:			
240 calories	140 calories from fat	15 g total fat	2 g saturated fat
0 mg cholesterol	240 mg sodium	25 g carbohydrates	11 g fiber
11 g sugar	7 g protein	1,317 mg potassium	101 mg calcium

1 head butter lettuce	1 TB. extra-virgin olive oil
$^1/_2$ cucumber	1 TB. balsamic vinegar
1 small green pepper	2 tsp. chia seeds
4 large tomatoes	$^1/_4$ tsp. sea salt
2 stalks (about $^1/_2$ lb.) broccoli	$^1/_4$ tsp. cracked black pepper
1 large avocado	

1. Wash butter lettuce leaves carefully and tear into 2-inch squares.

2. Dice cucumber, green pepper, and tomatoes.

3. Chop up broccoli. Remove end from avocado, cut in half, remove pit, and dice insides.

4. In a small bowl, combine extra-virgin olive oil and balsamic vinegar.

5. In a large bowl, place butter lettuce, diced ingredients, chia seeds, sea salt, and black pepper and toss.

6. Divide into bowls and serve.

 CHIA CAUTION

Choose your lettuces carefully. Iceberg lettuce, the longtime favorite in America, appears to be about as low in nutrition as a lettuce can manage to be. Butter lettuce and romaine lettuce are just two of many examples of more nutritious lettuces.

Kale Caesar Salad with Parmesan-Chia-Hemp Crisps

Caesar salad is famous for having a rich, smooth, delicious taste. Unfortunately, it usually gets that taste by including lots of cream, with calories and fat. Our version avoids all that and keeps the flavors without all the fat. The crisps can also be made with poppy seeds, sesame seeds, or other seeds for variety.

Yield:	Prep time:	Cook time:	Serving size:
2 cups salad plus 6 crisps	20 minutes	10 minutes	about $^1/_3$ cup salad plus 1 crisp

Each serving has:			
310 calories	250 calories from fat	27 g total fat	7 g saturated fat
75 mg cholesterol	390 mg sodium	7 g carbohydrates	1 g fiber
1 g sugar	11 g protein	147 mg potassium	318 mg calcium

$^1/_3$ cup freshly grated Parmesan cheese

1 TB. chia seeds

1 TB. hemp seeds

$^1/_4$ cup lemon juice

1 egg yolk

2 tsp. Dijon mustard

1 TB red wine vinegar

2 TB. chopped fresh garlic

Small tin anchovies

$^1/_2$ cup extra-virgin olive oil

1 bunch (about 9 oz.) kale

Sea salt

Cracked black pepper

1. Preheat the oven to 350°F.

2. On a silpat mat or parchment-lined sheet pan, place 6 $1^1/_2$-tablespoon mounds Parmesan cheese. Sprinkle mounds with chia seeds and hemp seeds and bake for 10 minutes or until golden brown. Set aside.

3. In a blender, place lemon juice, egg yolk, Dijon mustard, red wine vinegar, garlic, and anchovies and blend on emulsify setting, drizzling extra-virgin olive oil in until dressing is thick and creamy. Add remaining Parmesan cheese to incorporate. Set aside.

4. Wash kale and spin dry. Tear into bite-sized pieces, place in a medium salad bowl, and add dressing.

5. Serve in bowls with crisps on the side.

Chia and Hempseed Kale Chips

These chips have a rich, oily, satisfying flavor while having the nice crunch potato chips are famous for. They are far more nutritious than typical store-bought chips and provide a strong contribution to your daily chia goal.

Yield:	Prep time:	Cook time:	Serving size:
6 bowls chips	30 minutes	30 minutes in oven or 8 hours in dehydrator	1 bowl chips

Each serving has:			
250 calories	150 calories from fat	17 g total fat	5 g saturated fat
5 mg cholesterol	50 mg sodium	14 g carbohydrates	3 g fiber
2 g sugar	13 g protein	275 mg potassium	104 mg calcium

1 head (about 9 oz.) kale	1½ TB. sweet Thai chili sauce
8 cloves chopped garlic	2 Thai bird chiles
2 TB. whole dried shrimp	3 kaffir lime leaves, julienned thin
2 TB. coconut oil	1 cup shelled hemp seeds
3 TB. chia seeds	Sea salt
2 TB. nutritional yeast	Ground black pepper
¾ cup chia gel	

1. Preheat the oven to 275°F or preheat a dehydrator to 115°F.

2. Remove stem from kale, wash kale, and tear into bite-sized pieces. Peel garlic and chop fine. Set aside.

3. In a medium saucepan over medium heat, sauté shrimp in 1 tablespoon coconut oil until golden brown.

4. In a blender, place chia gel, chopped garlic, sweet Thai chile sauce, dried shrimp, Thai bird chilies, kaffir lime leaves, hemp seeds, sea salt to taste, black pepper to taste, and remaining 1 tablespoon coconut oil and blend on the purée setting until smooth. Season more with sea salt and black pepper as desired.

5. On a cookie sheet, spread kale and pour mixture generously over it.

6. Bake in the oven for 30 minutes or place in the dehydrator for 8 hours.

7. Put kale chips into bowls and serve.

Crispy Honey and Spice Chia Almonds

This snack combines several healthy snack foods into a tasty mix. You get the sweetness of honey and the nutty crunch of almonds.

Yield:	Prep time:	Cook time:	Serving size:
2 cups almonds	10 minutes	30 minutes	1/3 cup almonds

Each serving has:			
380 calories	260 calories from fat	29 g total fat	4.5 g saturated fat
10 mg cholesterol	30 mg sodium	24 g carbohydrates	8 g fiber
13 g sugar	11 g protein	355 mg potassium	161 mg calcium

2 TB. butter

1/4 cup honey

1 tsp. ground cinnamon

1/4 tsp. ground nutmeg

1/4 tsp. cayenne pepper

Sea salt

Ground black pepper

2 cups raw almonds, pecans, or cashews

3 TB. chia seeds

1. Preheat the oven to 350°F.

2. In a small saucepan over low heat, start melting butter and honey.

3. Add cinnamon, nutmeg, cayenne pepper, sea salt to taste, and black pepper to taste.

4. Once melted, turn off flame and stir in almonds and chia seeds with a rubber spatula until evenly coated.

5. On a cookie sheet, spread almonds. Bake until crunchy and caramelized, about 30 minutes.

6. Allow to cool and serve.

Strawberry-Chia Spread

The sweet flavor of fresh strawberries is enhanced with honey and made nutritionally richer with chia in this delicious recipe.

Yield:	Prep time:	Cook time:	Serving size:
about 5 TB. spread	20 minutes	1 hour	1 tsp. spread

Each serving has:			
35 calories	5 calories from fat	1 g total fat	0 g saturated fat
0 mg cholesterol	0 mg sodium	7 g carbohydrates	2 g fiber
5 g sugar	1 g protein	6 mg potassium	20 mg calcium

2 cups fresh strawberries	¼ cup chia seeds
1 cup water	¼ cup honey

1. Clean and slice strawberries.

2. In a medium pot, place strawberries, water, chia seeds, and honey and bring to a boil over high heat.

3. Reduce heat to medium and stir constantly until mixture has thickened and reduced in size by half.

4. Place spread a jar or other container and let cool for 1 hour.

5. Refrigerate for 5 hours to overnight before using. Serve spread on crackers or toast.

 FOOD FOR THOUGHT

As with many dishes based on fruit, strawberries aren't a big source of calories, but the sweeteners you might add to them are. This spread isn't as sweet as a jam and is quite healthy. Also, the sweeter and riper the strawberries you use, the less honey you'll need—allowing you to cut the calories in this dish while keeping the sweet and delicious flavor of the spread.

Carrots with Chia-Greek Yogurt Dip

Quick, handy snacks are crucial to eating well. Add some chia to Greek yogurt, and you have a tangy and creamy dip for veggies, such as carrots.

Yield:	Prep time:	Serving size:	
2 cups carrots plus $^1/_2$ cup Greek yogurt	5 minutes	1 cup carrots plus $^1/_4$ cup Greek yogurt	

Each serving has:			
290 calories	130 calories from fat	15 g total fat	9 g saturated fat
20 mg cholesterol	190 mg sodium	29 g carbohydrates	10 g fiber
14 g sugar	11 g protein	740 mg potassium	233 mg calcium

1 lb. carrots	1 cup Greek yogurt
2 TB. chia seeds	

1. Wash carrots. Quarter carrots lengthwise and chop into 1-inch spears.

2. In a small bowl, add chia seeds and Greek yogurt and stir.

3. Serve carrots on a plate with the bowl of yogurt dip.

Chia Seed Poppadums

For those who grew up on white bread or wheat bread, a poppadum is like a cross between bread and a tortilla chip. It tastes bready and crunchy but doesn't have the bulk of other breads. Poppadums are also often peppery and spicy, which makes them a good match for Indian curries and similar dishes. You'll improve your diet if you substitute moderate numbers of poppadums for slices of bread.

Yield:	Prep time:	Cook time:	Serving size:
6 (5-in.) poppadums	1 hour and 20 minutes	30 minutes	1 poppadum

Each serving has:			
60 calories	20 calories from fat	2 g total fat	0 g saturated fat
0 mg cholesterol	200 mg sodium	7 g carbohydrates	3 g fiber
2 g sugar	2 g protein	45 mg potassium	43 mg calcium

$1/2$ tsp. cumin seeds	2 cups vegetable broth
$1/4$ cup chia seeds	Sea salt
$1/4$ tsp. garlic powder	$1/4$ cup chickpea flour
$1/4$ tsp. ground black pepper	

1. In a small sauté pan on low heat, toast cumin seeds lightly to release oils.

2. Add chia seeds, garlic powder, black pepper, vegetable broth, and sea salt to taste and stir.

3. Remove from heat and set aside for about 45 minutes to 1 hour until it forms a thick gel.

4. Preheat the oven to 350°F.

5. Sift chickpea flour into wet mixture and fold in until combined well. Don't overmix.

6. On a cookie sheet, place mixture and roll out thin and evenly.

7. Bake for about 25 to 30 minutes until golden brown and crispy.

8. Let cool and serve.

Chia Energy Balls

These round little balls combine the richness and smoky complexity of raw chocolate, the smoothness of almond butter, the chewiness of coconut, and the sweetness of honey to make a snack that's fun to eat and nutritious.

Yield:	Prep time:	Serving size:	
20 (1-TB.) energy balls	45 minutes	2 energy balls	
Each serving has:			
230 calories	150 calories from fat	17 g total fat	8 g saturated fat
0 mg cholesterol	30 mg sodium	16 g carbohydrates	4 g fiber
9 g sugar	4 g protein	55 mg potassium	53 mg calcium

¹/₂ cup raw chocolate nibs	¹/₂ cup almond butter
¹/₂ cup shredded coconut	2 TB. honey
¹/₂ cup chia seeds	1 tsp. ground cinnamon

1. In a medium bowl, combine raw chocolate nibs, shredded coconut, chia seeds, almond butter, honey, and ground cinnamon, mixing thoroughly.

2. Place the bowl in the refrigerator and refrigerate for 30 minutes.

3. Roll dough into tablespoon-size balls.

4. Wrap or place energy balls in an airtight container and refrigerate until ready to eat. Energy balls are good up to 1 week.

 CHIA CAUTION

Most chocolate is made with a fair amount of butter or similar fat, and that's where most of the calories come from. Make sure you stick to raw chocolate, which is low in fat and calories

Chia Seed Granola

Granola is easy to make and endlessly flexible. This simple recipe creates a nicely chewy, slightly sweet granola that works well as a snack on the go.

Yield:	Prep time:	Cook time:	Serving size:
1 cup granola	10 minutes	15 minutes	$^1/_4$ cup granola

Each serving has:			
150 calories	60 calories from fat	6 g total fat	0 g saturated fat
21 mg cholesterol	0 mg sodium	21 g carbohydrates	4 g fiber
5 g sugar	4 g protein	10 mg potassium	45 mg calcium

1 cup oats	2 TB. chia seeds
1 tsp. ground cinnamon	1 TB. honey
$^1/_2$ tsp. ground nutmeg	1 TB. canola oil

1. Preheat the oven to 325°F. Put aluminum foil on a cookie sheet.

2. In a small bowl, combine oats, cinnamon, nutmeg, and chia seeds.

3. Add honey and canola oil and stir until oats are coated.

4. Spread granola mixture onto aluminum foil–covered cookie sheet.

5. Place the cookie sheet in the oven and bake for 10 minutes. Use a fork to stir and mix partly baked granola and place back in the oven to bake for 5 more minutes.

6. Allow granola to cool and serve.

Chocolate-Strawberry-Chia Chill

Strawberries dipped in chocolate are a food lover's delight. The fresh, delicious taste of strawberries and the complex richness of chocolate work well chilled, because the flavors come to life as the combination melts in your mouth.

Yield:	Prep time:	Serving size:	
1 cup chill	10 minutes	1/2 cup chill	
Each serving has:			
130 calories	20 calories from fat	2.5 g total fat	0 g saturated fat
0 mg cholesterol	85 mg sodium	27 g carbohydrates	6 g fiber
15 g sugar	3 g protein	298 mg potassium	136 mg calcium

1/3 cup unsweetened almond milk	1 TB. chia seeds
1 scoop chocolate whey powder	1 TB. cocoa powder
1/2 cup (about 10) frozen strawberries	Dash cinnamon
1 frozen banana	Dash chili powder

1. In a blender, place unsweetened almond milk, chocolate whey powder, strawberries, banana, chia seeds, cocoa powder, cinnamon, and chili powder and let sit for 5 minutes so chia seeds start to thicken mixture.

2. Blend on high until smooth.

3. Spoon into cups and serve.

 SEEDS OF CHANGE

Like so many chia recipes, this one is almost infinitely flexible. For instance, you can put bigger fruits such as strawberries in the mix that you blend and then pour it over smaller fruits like blueberries or pitted cherries for a rich mix of flavors, textures, and nutrition.

Dinners

Dinner is a big opportunity for cooking with chia. At least in Western cultures, dinner is the biggest meal of the day. Whether you were raised on dinners of fish sticks or duck a l'orange, what you eat at this time of day is significant.

Dinner is a time to get really creative with different foods and ingredients, including chia. As you know, chia seeds absorb water and expand in your stomach, so mixing some chia into your meals will help you control your appetite during a meal that tends to be heavy and prone to overindulgence.

Try experimenting with recipes where chia adds to the taste and texture of what you're eating. For example, the crab and chia recipe in this chapter lets you indulge in crab without having to break the bank, yet still feel full afterward.

While you may have days where you forget to consume chia early on, avoid loading chia into dinner to "catch up." Chia helps curb your appetite, which is great for meals during the day but not very helpful in the evenings. The focus on chia with dinner is moderation. Use a smaller amount of chia than you might earlier in the day to get the nutritional benefits of chia without overfilling yourself. And from the point of view of calories, all you want to do with chia at this point is stretch your meal a bit so you don't overeat.

In This Chapter

- Filling chia seafood dinners
- Pastas and stir-fries with chia
- Comfort foods, such as chia meatloaf
- Vegetarian and vegan chia main courses

Chia Crab Imperial

The light, tangy taste of crab; includes the richness of egg, the smoothness of mayonnaise rounding it out, and the spicy heat of Tabasco make this a fun and slightly spicy dish.

Yield:	Prep time:	Cook time:	Serving size:
2 cups crab	15 minutes	20 to 25 minutes	$^1/_2$ cup crab

Each serving has:			
350 calories	210 calories from fat	24 g total fat	4.5 g saturated fat
160 mg cholesterol	1,030 mg sodium	6 g carbohydrates	1 g fiber
0 g sugar	26 g protein	9.7 mg potassium	105 mg calcium

1 egg, lightly beaten	Juice and zest of $^1/_2$ lemon
$^1/_2$ cup light mayonnaise	$^1/_4$ tsp. sea salt
2 tsp. Old Bay seasoning	$^1/_4$ tsp. cracked black pepper
$^1/_4$ cup chopped parsley	4 tsp. chia seeds
Tabasco sauce	1 lb. crab meat

1. Preheat the oven to 375°F.

2. In a medium oven-proof bowl, mix egg, mayonnaise, Old Bay seasoning, parsley, tabasco sauce to taste, lemon juice, lemon zest, sea salt, black pepper, and chia seeds, blending well.

3. Pick through crab meat to make sure there aren't any shells in it.

4. Add crab meat to bowl and fold in gently without breaking up crab meat lumps.

5. Place in the oven and bake for 20 to 25 minutes, or until golden brown and set.

6. Serve in cups, on lettuce leaves, or on a buttered ramekin, or use to stuff your favorite fish, shellfish, mushrooms, or peppers.

Chia Meatloaf

This meatloaf combines the rich taste of ground meat with the spicy hit of garlic and onion. Eggs, oatmeal, and chia add a smooth consistency and hold it all together.

Yield:	Prep time:	Cook time:	Serving size:
1 (9×5-in.) meatloaf	30 minutes	25 minutes	1 slice meatloaf

Each serving has:			
360 calories	150 calories from fat	16 g total fat	6 g saturated fat
180 mg cholesterol	1,500 mg sodium	20 g carbohydrates	5 g fiber
3 g sugar	31 g protein	482 mg potassium	73 mg calcium

1 lb. ground beef (90/10), turkey, pork, or other ground meat

2 eggs

2 TB. chia seeds

$^3/_4$ cup oatmeal

$^1/_4$ cup garlic, chopped

$^1/_4$ cup yellow onion, minced

$^1/_8$ cup celery, minced

$^1/_8$ cup carrot, minced

$^1/_4$ tsp. sea salt

$^1/_4$ tsp. cracked black pepper

3 TB. fresh thyme, chopped

$^1/_4$ cup sweet soy sauce

1. Preheat the oven to 375°F.

2. In a large bowl, mix ground beef, eggs, chia seeds, and oatmeal.

3. Fold in garlic, yellow onion, celery, and carrot. Season with sea salt and black pepper.

4. Place meatloaf mixture in a 9×5-inch oven-safe glass or metal loaf pan and bake for 10 minutes.

5. Remove from the oven, brush on sweet soy sauce, and place back in oven until meatloaf is browned on top and soy sauce has thickened and is bubbling, about 15 minutes.

6. Let cool for 10 minutes and serve.

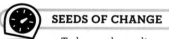 **SEEDS OF CHANGE**

To lower the sodium content of this recipe, consider using low-sodium soy sauce.

Coconut, Pecan, and Chia-Crusted Salmon

Salmon has a rich, meaty taste—and it doesn't taste or smell "fishy" in the usual and sometimes off-putting sense. This recipe adds eggs, breadcrumbs, and tangy coconut for additional flavor and texture.

Yield:	Prep time:	Cook time:	Serving size:
4 (6-oz.) pieces crusted salmon	30 minutes	25 minutes	1 piece crusted salmon

Each serving has:			
700 calories	430 calories from fat	48 g total fat	19 g saturated fat
225 mg cholesterol	420 mg sodium	30 g carbohydrates	7 g fiber
4 g sugar	35 g protein	486 mg potassium	106 mg calcium

3 eggs, whipped	1 cup unsweetened coconut flakes
$1/4$ tsp. sea salt	$2/3$ cup pecans, finely chopped
$1/4$ tsp. cracked black pepper	2 TB. chia seeds
1 cup breadcrumbs or gluten-free breadcrumbs	2 tsp. garlic powder
	4 (4-oz.) pieces salmon

1. Preheat the oven to 375°F.

2. In a medium bowl, pour in eggs and season with pinch sea salt and pinch black pepper.

3. In another medium bowl, mix breadcrumbs, unsweetened coconut flakes, pecans, chia seeds, and garlic powder. Season with remaining sea salt and remaining black pepper.

4. Dredge each piece of salmon in egg mixture. Place in breadcrumb mixture and cover, pressing down so breading sticks to all sides.

5. Place on a 9×13-inch or larger sheet pan and put in the oven for 8 to 10 minutes, until salmon is crispy on the edges.

6. Serve.

 CHIA CAUTION

This recipe does pack a caloric punch, but it's full of omega-3 fatty acids, as well as healthy antioxidants. This isn't an entrée you should eat daily—or maybe even weekly if you're dieting—but it's a good treat once a month.

Baked Ziti with Chia and Ricotta Cheese

The combination of the rich flavor of pasta and cheese is a worldwide favorite. Baking them together with the tangy taste of tomatoes makes a dish that most people find hard to resist.

Yield:	Prep time:	Cook time:	Serving size:
8 slices ziti	30 minutes	35 minutes	1 (2×2$^1/_2$-in.) slice

Each serving has:			
430 calories	160 calories from fat	18 g total fat	8 g saturated fat
45 mg cholesterol	950 mg sodium	44 g carbohydrates	4 g fiber
11 g sugar	22 g protein	16 mg potassium	263 mg calcium

$^1/_2$ lb. uncooked ziti

4 cups marinara sauce

$^1/_2$ lb. low-fat ricotta cheese, drained

4 tsp. chia seeds

$^1/_2$ bunch (about 3 sprigs) fresh basil, snipped

Sea salt

Cracked black pepper

$^1/_2$ lb. fresh mozzarella, sliced thin

$^1/_2$ cup grated sharp provolone cheese

1. Preheat the oven to 400°F.

2. Fill a large pot of salted water and bring to a boil over high heat.

3. Add ziti, stir, and cook until al dente, about 9 to 12 minutes. Drain ziti and set aside.

4. In a medium saucepot over medium-high heat, heat marinara sauce to a simmer. Add low-fat ricotta cheese, chia seeds, basil, sea salt to taste, and black pepper to taste and stir.

5. In an 8×10-inch oven-safe glass dish, spread a thin layer of sauce on the bottom.

6. Layer half of ziti over sauce.

7. Cover with ¼ pound mozzarella cheese and ¼ cup sharp provolone cheese.

8. Spread 1 cup sauce over cheese in an even layer.

9. Add rest of ziti, remaining ¼ pound mozzarella cheese, and remaining ¼ cup sharp provolone cheese. Spoon final layer of sauce over top.

10. Place dish in the oven and bake, uncovered, until golden brown and bubbling, about 35 minutes.

11. Allow baked ziti to sit for 10 minutes before slicing and serving.

Chia Stir-Fry Beef with Broccoli

The rich flavor of beef and the slightly spicy taste of broccoli are a delicious combination, recognized by beef and broccoli dishes in many different cultures. This one adds a bit of onion and garlic for bite.

Yield:	Prep time:	Cook time:	Serving size:
$1^1/_2$ lb. stir-fry	15 minutes	10 minutes	$^1/_4$ lb. stir-fry

Each serving has:			
250 calories	120 calories from fat	14 g total fat	3.5 g saturated fat
50 mg cholesterol	660 mg sodium	8 g carbohydrates	2 g fiber
1 g sugar	23 g protein	44 mg potassium	32 mg calcium

1 lb. sirloin beef tips, sliced into $^1/_4$-in.-wide strips	2 cloves garlic
$1^1/_2$ TB. cornstarch	1 TB. chia seeds
$^1/_4$ tsp. sea salt	1 TB. flaxseeds
$^1/_4$ tsp. cracked black pepper	1 TB sesame seeds
$^1/_4$ tsp. garlic powder	3 TB. reduced-sodium soy sauce
3 TB. vegetable oil	$^1/_2$ tsp. ground ginger
1 cup frozen broccoli florets	$^1/_3$ cup water
1 small onion, sliced	

1. In a medium bowl, coat sirloin beef tips in cornstarch, sea salt, black pepper, and garlic powder.

2. In a large skillet or wok over medium high heat, add 2 tablespoons vegetable oil, place coated beef tips, and stir-fry until beef is brown on all sides, about 6 minutes.

3. Remove beef tips and transfer to a medium bowl. Wrap the bowl in tinfoil to keep warm, and set aside.

4. Add remaining 1 tablespoon vegetable oil to the skillet or wok. Add broccoli florets, onion, garlic, chia seeds, flaxseeds, and sesame seeds and stir-fry over medium-high heat until broccoli is just tender and garlic is pale golden, about 2 minutes.

5. Add reduced-sodium soy sauce, ginger, and water and bring to a boil over high heat. Add beef tips and cook, stirring, until sauce is thickened, about 2 minutes.

6. Serve over a bed of rice.

Almond and Chia-Encrusted Chicken Breast

This nutty chicken dish is complemented by the bite of mustard and the subtle spiciness of grapeseed oil.

Yield:	Prep time:	Cook time:	Serving size:
4 (3-oz.) chicken breasts	15 minutes	10 minutes	1 chicken breast

Each serving has:			
380 calories	220 calories from fat	25 g total fat	2.5 g saturated fat
75 mg cholesterol	240 mg sodium	7 g carbohydrates	4 g fiber
1 g sugar	33 g protein	464 mg potassium	86 mg calcium

4 (3-oz.) boneless, skinless chicken breasts	4 tsp. chia seeds
2 egg whites	1 tsp. dried parsley
1 heaping tsp. ground mustard	$1/4$ tsp. sea salt
1 cup almond meal	$1/4$ tsp. ground black pepper
2 TB. grapeseed oil	

1. Cut chicken breasts in half to flatten out.

2. In a large bowl, add egg whites and ground mustard and whisk until incorporated.

3. In a small food processor or blender, add almond meal, grapeseed oil, and chia seeds and pulse until smooth.

4. Pour meal-seed mixture onto a flat plate and sprinkle with parsley, sea salt and black pepper. Mix with a fork to incorporate evenly.

5. Heat a large nonstick pan on medium to high heat. Dip each chicken piece into egg-mustard mixture. Lay chicken flat o the plate with meal-seed mixture, press down firmly, and flip over until both sides are covered.

6. Place chicken in the hot pan and cook for 3 to 4 minutes per side or until center is no longer pink.

7. Serve. This dish is great with a simple salad of thinly sliced cabbage and a drizzle of red wine vinegar.

Chia Jambalaya

Jambalaya is a Creole-Cajun dish famous for being spicy and delicious, with lots of flavors. This vegetarian version uses chia as a source of extra nutrients.

Yield:	Prep time:	Cook time:	Serving size:
6 bowls jambalaya	15 minutes	1 hour and 15 minutes	1 bowl jambalaya

Each serving has:			
290 calories	80 calories from fat	9 g total fat	1 g saturated fat
0 mg cholesterol	500 mg sodium	43 g carbohydrates	6 g fiber
7 g sugar	11 g protein	170 mg potassium	70 mg calcium

1 medium green bell pepper	2 TB. chia seeds
3 celery stalks	1 tsp. paprika
1 large onion	1 tsp. dried oregano
3 cloves garlic	1 tsp. dried basil
1 (8-oz.) package vegan sausage	$1/2$ tsp. dried thyme
$2^1/2$ cups water	1 tsp. cayenne
1 cup uncooked brown rice	1 tsp. sea salt
2 TB. olive oil	
1 (28-oz.) can diced tomatoes, with liquid	

1. Dice green bell pepper and celery, chop onion stalks, and mince garlic.

2. Slice sausage into links ¼ inch thick.

3. In a medium saucepan over medium heat, bring water to a simmer.

4. Stir in brown rice and cook for 35 minutes or until water is absorbed.

5. In a large skillet over medium-high heat, heat 1 tablespoon olive oil. Add vegan sausages and brown evenly, about 10 minutes.

6. Add remaining 1 tablespoon olive oil to the skillet. Add onion and sauté on medium-high until onion is softened, about 5 minutes. Add green bell pepper, celery, garlic, and tomatoes and sauté until all are browned, about 10 minutes.

7. Add chia seeds, paprika, oregano, basil, thyme, cayenne, and sea salt and bring to a simmer. Reduce heat to low, cover, and simmer gently for 15 minutes.

8. Combine sausage mixture with rice, toss, and serve.

 FOOD FOR THOUGHT

The great thing about so many vegan and vegetarian dishes is that you can always toss in a little meat, cheese, or dairy for friends who think that "if it's meatless, it isn't a meal." Even if you're in that camp yourself, use vegan and vegetarian recipes as a starting point at first and then make more of your meals vegan and vegetarian over time.

Black Bean, Hemp, and Chia Patties

Trying to create exact substitutes for meat is a tricky process. Reproducing the taste and mouth-feel of a slightly greasy hamburger is really hard to do well with vegetables. In our opinion, it's better to create vegan and vegetarian food that serves the same function in recipes as meat but has its own unique and interesting taste and flavor. These black bean patties have the rich and cool flavor of beans, held together with hemp and chia.

Yield:	Prep time:	Cook time:	Serving size:
6 patties	15 minutes	1 hour	1 patty
Each serving has:			
410 calories	140 calories from fat	15 g total fat	2.5 g saturated fat
0 mg cholesterol	340 mg sodium	51 g carbohydrates	7 g fiber
6 g sugar	18 g protein	421 mg potassium	87 mg calcium

2 tsp. coconut oil	$^1/_2$ tsp. sea salt
$^1/_2$ medium yellow onion	2 tsp. paprika powder
1 red bell pepper	$^1/_4$ tsp. chipotle powder
4 large cloves garlic	$^1/_4$ tsp. cayenne powder
10 Roma tomatoes	2 tsp. miso paste
$1^1/_2$ cups cooked black beans	1 cup cooked brown rice
1 cup hemp seeds	$^1/_3$ cup quinoa flakes
6 tsp. chia seeds	

1. Dice onion and red bell pepper and mince garlic.

2. In a medium frying pan over medium heat, heat 1 teaspoon coconut oil. Add onion and garlic and cook about 5 minutes.

3. Add red bell pepper and cook for 5 more minutes.

4. Add Roma tomatoes, black beans, hemp seeds, chia seeds, sea salt, paprika powder, chipotle powder, and cayenne powder, reduce heat to low, and cook for 2 minutes.

5. Transfer to a large bowl and add miso paste, beans, brown rice, and quinoa flakes. Knead mixture together.

6. Cover and place in the refrigerator for 30 minutes. Quinoa and chia will swell and absorb the excess water.

7. Remove from the refrigerator and form mixture into 6 patties.

8. In a medium frying pan over medium heat, warm remaining 1 teaspoon coconut oil. Add three patties and cook for 4 to 5 minutes on one side or until browned. Repeat for remaining patties.

9. Serve.

Vegan Chia Paella

Paella is famous as a rice dish with saffron and lots of fish. This version substitutes vegetables to create a rich mix of flavors.

Yield:	Prep time:	Cook time:	Serving size:
6 bowls paella	10 minutes	30 minutes	1 bowl paella

Each serving has:			
220 calories	35 calories from fat	4 g total fat	.5 g saturated fat
0 mg cholesterol	290 mg sodium	42 g carbohydrates	8 g fiber
10 g sugar	7 g protein	624 mg potassium	65 mg calcium

1 medium onion

3 cloves garlic

1 green bell pepper

1 red bell pepper

6 ripe medium tomatoes

1 (14-oz.) can artichoke hearts

1 bunch (about 6 sprigs) fresh parsley

2 tsp. extra-virgin olive oil

1 (15-oz.) can vegetable broth

$^3/_4$ cup uncooked quick brown rice

1 tsp. saffron

$^1/_2$ tsp. dried thyme

2 TB. chia seeds

1 cup water

$1^1/_2$ cups green peas

$^1/_4$ tsp. sea salt

$^1/_4$ tsp. black pepper

1. Chop onion and mince garlic.

2. Cut green bell pepper and red bell pepper into 2-inch strips. Dice tomatoes. Drain artichoke hearts and chop into chunks. Chop fresh parsley.

3. In a large skillet over medium heat, heat extra-virgin olive oil. Add onion and garlic and sauté for 5 minutes.

4. Add green and red bell pepper and sauté for 5 more minutes.

5. Add tomatoes, vegetable broth, brown rice, saffron, thyme, chia seeds, and water, turn up heat to high, and bring to a simmer. Reduce heat to low, cover, and simmer gently for 10 minutes.

6. Stir in artichoke hearts and green peas.

7. Add sea salt and black pepper and a little water if needed for the rice and cook over low heat for 5 more minutes.

8. Serve from the pan.

Macaroni and Chia Cheese

The chewy texture of macaroni and the delicious taste of cheese are a longtime favorite. Using vegetarian substitutes captures the same spicy smoothness, while adding chia makes the whole thing more nutritious.

Yield:	Cook time:	Serving size:	
6 bowls macaroni and cheese	45 minutes	1 bowl macaroni and cheese	

Each serving has:			
590 calories	240 calories from fat	27 g total fat	4.5 g saturated fat
0 mg cholesterol	910 mg sodium	68 g carbohydrates	9 g fiber
3 g sugar	22 g protein	601 mg potassium	35 mg calcium

4 cups water	3 TB. soy sauce
4 cups elbow macaroni	2 tsp. garlic powder
$1/2$ cup vegan margarine	$1/8$ tsp. turmeric
$1/2$ cup all-purpose flour	$1/4$ cup vegetable oil
2 TB. chia seeds	1 cup yeast flakes
$1/2$ tsp. sea salt	

1. Preheat the oven to 350°F.

2. Pour 2 cups water into a medium saucepan and bring to a boil over high heat. Add elbow macaroni and cook until springy, about 10 minutes. Put into a casserole dish and set aside.

3. In a medium saucepan over low heat, melt vegan margarine. Whisk in all-purpose flour, about 5 minutes.

4. Raise heat to medium and whisk flour and margarine until bubbly, about 5 more minutes.

5. Raise heat to high and whisk in remaining 2 cups water, chia seeds, sea salt, soy sauce, garlic powder, turmeric, vegetable oil, and yeast flakes. Bring to a boil and cook for about 5 minutes.

6. Pour mixture over macaroni in the casserole dish.

7. Place the casserole dish in the oven and bake for 15 minutes.

8. Broil for 5 minutes, until top is crispy. Remove from the oven and serve.

"Beef" and Chia Stroganoff

This is a great way to try a recipe that uses a beef substitute. The result is a rich, delicious, tangy dish that tastes a lot like traditional beef stroganoff.

Yield:	Prep time:	Cook time:	Serving size:
6 plates stroganoff	5 minutes	30 minutes	1 plate stroganoff

Each serving has:			
400 calories	60 calories from fat	7 g total fat	2 g saturated fat
5 mg cholesterol	950 mg sodium	64 g carbohydrates	8 g fiber
5 g sugar	20 g protein	283 mg potassium	86 mg calcium

$^1/_2$ lb. mushrooms	Pinch garlic powder
4 cups water	$^1/_4$ tsp. black pepper
1 lb. egg noodles	$^1/_4$ tsp. sea salt
1 TB. vegetable oil	2 TB. chia seeds
1 medium onion	4 oz. plain Greek yogurt
1 lb. vegan burger crumbles	$^3/_4$ cup white wine (optional)
1 (10-oz.) can mushroom gravy	

1. Slice mushrooms.

2. In a medium pot over high heat, bring water to a boil.

3. Reduce heat to medium, add egg noodles, and cook until springy, about 7 to 8 minutes. Drain.

4. In a large skillet over medium heat, add vegetable oil. Add onion and brown, about 5 minutes.

5. Add vegan burger crumbles, mushroom gravy, garlic powder, black pepper, sea salt, chia seeds, Greek yogurt, and white wine (if using), cover, and cook on medium for 15 minutes.

6. Pour sauce over noodles and serve.

Chickpea Salad Wrap with Chia

Chickpeas have a rich, satisfying flavor, which makes them a good replacement for meat. This wrap is a good centerpiece for a light dinner, and you can use any leftovers for lunch and snacks.

Yield:	Prep time:	Serving size:	
3 wraps	20 minutes	1 wrap	
Each serving has:			
180 calories	35 calories from fat	4 g total fat	0 g saturated fat
0 mg cholesterol	140 mg sodium	27 g carbohydrates	6 g fiber
2 g sugar	8 g protein	340 mg potassium	67 mg calcium

1 (15-oz.) can chickpeas	1 TB. chia seeds
1/2 fresh lemon	1/2 tsp. mustard powder
2 stalks celery	1/4 cup pecans
1/2 small red onion	1/4 tsp. sea salt
1 large kosher dill pickle	1/4 tsp. black pepper
2 TB. fresh dill	3 pita pockets
1 garlic clove	

1. Drain chickpeas and mash them in a small bowl with a fork. Squeeze in juice from lemon.

2. Dice celery, red onion, and kosher dill pickle and add to chickpeas. Mince dill and garlic and add to chickpeas.

3. Add chia seeds, mustard powder, pecans, sea salt, and black pepper and stir until flavors are thoroughly mixed, about 2 to 3 minutes.

4. Stuff mixture into pita pockets and serve.

Chia Lasagna

This lasagna is rich, with the smooth flavor of noodles and the tangy taste of tomatoes.

Yield:	Prep time:	Cook time:	Serving size:
8 (1¹/₄-in.) squares lasagna	10 minutes	2 hours and 5 minutes	1 square lasagna

Each serving has:			
340 calories	130 calories from fat	14 g total fat	1.5 g saturated fat
0 mg cholesterol	770 mg sodium	41 g carbohydrates	9 g fiber
5 g sugar	17 g protein	42 mg potassium	280 mg calcium

2 lb. spinach leaves	6 tsp. chia seeds
1 lb. soft tofu	2 TB. lemon juice
1 lb. firm tofu	3 tsp. minced fresh basil
¹/₄ cup soy milk	4 cups tomato sauce
1 TB. granulated sugar	¹/₂ lb. lasagna noodles
¹/₂ tsp. garlic powder	

1. Preheat the oven to 350°F.

2. Wash spinach leaves carefully and tear into small pieces.

3. In a blender on slow speed, combine soft tofu, firm tofu, soy milk, sugar, garlic powder, chia seeds, lemon juice, basil, and chopped spinach leaves.

4. In a casserole dish, cover bottom with 1 cup tomato sauce. Layer in ¹/₃ of lasagna noodles and ¹/₃ of tofu mixture. Repeat layers until everything is used.

5. Place in the oven and bake for 2 hours. Test with a fork; it's done when the fork goes in and comes out dry.

6. Broil for 5 minutes to make the top crispy. Remove from the oven and serve.

 SEEDS OF CHANGE

This lasagna also serves as a good base for vegetables such as carrots or cucumbers. Learn how to make the lasagna and then experiment with additional ingredients to make it your own.

Roasted Peppers and Pasta with Chia

In this pasta, tangy, rich red peppers combine with cool pesto and crunchy walnuts.

Yield:	Prep time:	Cook time:	Serving size:
3 bowls pasta	5 minutes	10 to 12 minutes	1 bowl pasta

Each serving has:			
560 calories	260 calories from fat	29 g total fat	3.5 g saturated fat
0 mg cholesterol	0 mg sodium	62 g carbohydrates	4 g fiber
7 g sugar	10 g protein	269 mg potassium	21 mg calcium

2 large red peppers

1 bunch (about 6 sprigs) fresh basil

1 bunch (about 6 sprigs) fresh
　parsley

1 clove garlic

4 cups water

$1/2$ lb. dry pasta

$1/3$ cup walnuts

$1/4$ cup olive oil

1. Chop red peppers, basil, and parsley. Mince garlic.

2. In a large saucepan over high heat, bring water to a boil, about 5 minutes.

3. Reduce heat to medium, add dry pasta, and cook until tender, about 5 to 7 minutes. Drain.

4. In a food processor on slow speed, mix walnuts and olive oil for about 1 minute.

5. Add walnut-oil pesto to noodles and toss.

6. Serve.

Spaghetti Squash with Chia

Rich, crisp spaghetti squash has a texture that allows you to use it as a substitute for pasta and is filling enough to help you not miss meat much. This recipe uses jarred spaghetti sauce to allow you to concentrate on the spaghetti squash, but feel free to make your own sauce.

Yield:	Prep time:	Cook time:	Serving size:
2 bowls spaghetti squash	5 minutes	45 minutes	1 bowl spaghetti squash

Each serving has:			
420 calories	80 calories from fat	9 g total fat	1.5 g saturated fat
0 mg cholesterol	600 mg sodium	89 g carbohydrates	5 g fiber
3 g sugar	11 g protein	1,239 mg potassium	319 mg calcium

1 (5-lb.) spaghetti squash	1/4 tsp. black pepper
1 tsp. olive oil	1 (8-oz.) jar spaghetti sauce
1/4 tsp. sea salt	2 TB. chia seeds

1. Preheat the oven to 350°F.

2. Cut end off spaghetti squash, cut squash in half lengthwise, and scoop out seeds.

3. Brush inner surface of spaghetti squash with olive oil and sprinkle with sea salt and black pepper.

4. Place spaghetti squash halves face down on a baking sheet lined with aluminum foil and roast for 45 minutes. Squash is done when you can scrape strands out with a fork.

5. During last 15 minutes of cooking squash, pour spaghetti sauce into a medium saucepan and add chia seeds. Bring to a simmer over medium heat, about 10 minutes. Turn off heat.

6. Remove squash from the oven and let cool for 5 minutes.

7. Scrape out squash flesh into two bowls.

8. Pour the spaghetti sauce-chia mixture over squash strands and serve.

 FOOD FOR THOUGHT

Spaghetti squash is a many-splendored base for a lot of recipes that normally use pasta. If you're going gluten free or just trying to reduce the amount of grain in your diet, spaghetti squash can be your friend.

CHAPTER 19

Side Dishes

Side dishes extend or round out a full meal. A main course, a side dish, and a vegetable really makes you feel like you've been fed, even if the portions are quite moderate. Add in a small dessert, such as fruit with a bit of yogurt, and you'll feel like you've had a feast.

Side dishes present an excellent way to add chia to your meal. They tend to be a bit more creative than main and vegetable dishes, making them more adaptable to addition or modification. Chia seeds are a perfect way to do it.

As you seek to eat a healthier diet, you can even change the balance somewhat. For example, in a meal, double the vegetable serving, or add a second vegetable, and cut the main course—usually centered around beef, chicken, or fish, if you're like most—in half. This lets you increase the side dish by a third or so. You'll be surprised by how full you feel, and both your nutritional balance and your bank balance will likely be much better (after all, meat is almost always the most expensive part of a meal).

Use the side dishes in this chapter as is and as an inspiration for your own efforts.

In This Chapter

- Substantial sides including chia, such as rice pilaf, sautéed kale, and cole slaw
- Potato salad and hummus, chia style
- Carrots, cucumbers, and avocado with chia

SEEDS OF CHANGE

Consider making your side dish your main dish. You can do this by extending it with something more that feels substantial, such as small chunks of some kind of meat, tempeh, or vegetables. You can even take the dish that was going to be your main course, cut the size by two thirds, and cut it into what was going to be your side dish.

Sautéed Kale with Chia, Lemon, Garlic, and Parmesan

Kale has a rich, exotic, grassy flavor that may take children—and some adults—a little getting used to. But pairing it with lemon, garlic, and Parmesan cheese makes it only too easy to like.

Yield:	Prep time:	Cook time:	Serving size:
4 bowls kale	8 minutes	7 minutes	1 bowl kale

Each serving has:			
180 calories	120 calories from fat	14 g total fat	3 g saturated fat
5 mg cholesterol	190 mg sodium	10 g carbohydrates	3 g fiber
10 g sugar	5 g protein	325 mg potassium	183 mg calcium

3 TB. extra-virgin olive oil	4 tsp. chia seeds
4 cloves chopped garlic	$1/4$ tsp. sea salt
1 bunch kale, washed, drained, and chopped small	$1/4$ tsp. cracked black pepper
Water	2 TB. fresh lemon juice
Crushed red pepper flakes	3 TB. fresh grated Parmesan cheese

1. In a large sauté pan over medium heat, heat extra-virgin olive oil. Stir in garlic and sauté until golden brown.

2. Add kale, splash of water, crushed red pepper flakes, chia seeds, sea salt, and black pepper and stir.

3. When kale is wilted and cooked down, add lemon juice and stir well.

4. Remove from heat, put into bowls, sprinkle ¾ tablespoon of fresh grated Parmesan cheese over each, and serve.

Saffron Rice and Chia Pilaf

The warm and—to many Westernized palates—somewhat exotic flavor of saffron brings this rice and vegetable dish to life.

Yield:	Prep time:	Cook time:	Serving size:
6 bowls rice	20 minutes	40 minutes	1 bowl rice

Each serving has:			
150 calories	45 calories from fat	5 g total fat	2.5 g saturated fat
10 mg cholesterol	540 mg sodium	21 g carbohydrates	3 g fiber
5 g sugar	4 g protein	98 mg potassium	33 mg calcium

3 cups chicken broth

1 shallot, minced

$1/2$ cup roasted red bell pepper, diced, peeled, and deseeded

2 TB. butter

$1/4$ tsp. sea salt

$1/4$ tsp. cracked black pepper

$1^1/2$ cups long-grain rice

4 tsp. chia seeds

2 tsp. lemon zest and juice

Pinch saffron bloomed in lemon zest and juice

1 bay leaf

1 cup frozen peas, thawed and rinsed

2 TB. currants, pistachios, or chopped almonds (optional)

1. Preheat the oven to 350°F.

2. In a small saucepan over medium heat, bring chicken broth to a simmer.

3. In a medium saucepan over medium heat, cook shallot and roasted red bell pepper in butter until translucent.

4. Add sea salt, black pepper, and long-grain rice, stirring to coat in butter. Continue to stir rice until golden brown with a nutty aroma.

5. Add cooked chicken broth, chia seeds, lemon zest and juice, saffron, and bay leaf and bring to a boil over high heat.

6. Give pilaf a good stir and place a white kitchen towel over top of saucepan. Place a lid on top of the towel, folding the excess over the top of the lid.

7. Place the covered saucepan in the oven and bake for 15 minutes or until rice is puffy and almost all liquid is absorbed. Remove from the oven and rest for 10 minutes before removing the lid.

8. Stir in peas and fluff pilaf with a fork. Garnish with currants, pistachios, or almonds (if using) and serve.

 CHIA CAUTION

Be careful when you put the towel on top of your saucepan. It will be absorbing steam and will get quite hot for a while. Handle the dry edges of the towel and use the back of your hand to quickly check the temperature of the wet parts before grabbing it.

Classic Potato Salad with Dill Pickle-Chia Relish

This version of a picnic classic adds crunchy celery and tangy onion to the savory flavor of potatoes. Including chia seeds heightens the nutritional benefits of the dish and helps people feel comfortably full hours after eating it.

Yield:	Prep time:	Cook time:	Serving size:
8 bowls potato salad	45 minutes	20 to 30 minutes	1 bowl potato salad

Each serving has:			
340 calories	220 calories from fat	24 g total fat	3.5 g saturated fat
65 mg cholesterol	450 mg sodium	26 g carbohydrates	4 g fiber
2 g sugar	5 g protein	640 mg potassium	41 mg calcium

3 Idaho potatoes, rinsed	1/4 cup dill pickle relish
2 large eggs	1/2 tsp. garlic powder
Sea salt	1/2 tsp. celery salt
Ground black pepper	1/4 cup chives, sliced thin
1 TB. cider vinegar	1 TB. Dijon mustard
1/4 cup onion, diced small	1/4 cup mayonnaise
1/4 cup celery, diced small	2 TB. chia seeds

1. In a large pot of salted water, place Idaho potatoes and bring to a boil over high heat. Once boiling, cook potatoes for about 15 minutes or until fork tender but still firm. Drain and cool.

2. Cut cooled potatoes into a medium dice. You can peel or not peel potatoes before dicing them, depending on your preference.

3. In a small saucepan, place eggs and cover with cold water. Add sea salt to taste, black pepper to taste, and cider vinegar and bring to a boil over high heat.

4. Cover saucepan and remove from heat, leaving eggs to slowly cook for about 13 to 15 minutes. Shock the eggs by dropping them in ice water and then peel and chop.

5. Combine diced potatoes, chopped eggs, onion, celery, dill pickle relish, garlic powder, celery salt, chives, Dijon mustard, mayonnaise, and chia seeds.

6. Refrigerate potato salad until chilled and ready to serve.

SEEDS OF CHANGE

To peel eggs, shock them with cold water as described in the recipe. You then roll them in all dimensions and directions on a cutting board, which cracks the shell into many small pieces. After you do this, the shell is easy to remove.

Chia-Apple Cole Slaw

This perennial favorite combines tangy vinegar, rich mayonnaise, and sweet honey.

Yield:	Prep time:	Serving size:	
4 cups cole slaw	20 minutes	$^1/_2$ cup cole slaw	

Each serving has:			
140 calories	110 calories from fat	12 g total fat	1.5 g saturated fat
5 mg cholesterol	130 mg sodium	7 g carbohydrates	2 g fiber
4 g sugar	1 g protein	174 mg potassium	66 mg calcium

3 cups shredded yellow cabbage

1 cup shredded purple cabbage, soaked and drained 3 times in ice water

1 carrot, shredded

$^1/_3$ cup mayonnaise

$1^1/_2$ TB. cider vinegar

2 TB. extra-virgin olive oil

$1^1/_2$ TB. honey or to taste

1 shallot, minced

$^1/_4$ cup chopped Italian flat-leaf parsley

2 TB. chia seeds

$^1/_4$ tsp. sea salt

$^1/_4$ tsp. cracked black pepper

1. In a large bowl, place yellow cabbage, purple cabbage, and carrot.

2. In a smaller bowl, whisk together mayonnaise, cider vinegar, extra-virgin olive oil, honey, shallot, Italian flat-leaf parsley, chia seeds, sea salt, and black pepper.

3. Pour mixture over cabbage and carrots and toss until thoroughly coated and mixed well.

4. Refrigerate cole slaw until ready to serve.

Maple-Glazed Carrots with Chia

Carrots are often regarded as somewhat boring, but they actually have a natural sweetness. In this dish, maple syrup enhances this natural flavor.

Yield:	Prep time:	Cook time:	Serving size:
4 cups carrots	10 minutes	15 to 20 minutes	about $1/2$ cup carrots

Each serving has:			
80 calories	30 calories from fat	3.5 g total fat	2 g saturated fat
10 mg cholesterol	100 mg sodium	12 g carbohydrates	2 g fiber
8 g sugar	1 g protein	2 mg potassium	29 mg calcium

$1^1/_2$ lb. baby carrots, or large carrots sliced $1/4$ in. on bias

$1/8$ cup maple syrup

2 TB. unsalted butter

$1/3$ cup vegetable broth

1 TB. chia seeds

$1/4$ tsp. sea salt

$1/4$ tsp. cracked black pepper

1 TB. fresh-squeezed orange juice

$1/2$ tsp. orange zest

1. In a medium sauté pan over medium heat, place baby carrots, maple syrup, unsalted butter, vegetable broth, chia seeds, sea salt, and black pepper and bring to a boil.

2. Reduce heat to a simmer and add orange juice and orange zest.

3. Stir occasionally, until carrots are tender. Continue simmering, uncovered, until cooking liquid is reduced to a syrupy glaze, about 13 minutes.

4. Spoon onto plates and serve.

Chia, Chickpea, and Tahini Hummus

Chickpeas have a savory, almost meaty flavor, especially when made into a spicy hummus. Garlic adds to the flavor of this delicious dish, and chia adds nutrition.

Yield:	Prep time:	Serving size:	
1 cup hummus	15 minutes	about $^1/_4$ cup hummus	

Each serving has:			
190 calories	130 calories from fat	14 g total fat	2 g saturated fat
0 mg cholesterol	85 mg sodium	13 g carbohydrates	3 g fiber
1 g sugar	5 g protein	162 mg potassium	56 mg calcium

$^3/_4$ cup chickpeas, cooked and drained (or canned chickpeas, rinsed and drained)

$^1/_4$ cup fresh-squeezed lemon juice

3 cloves garlic

3 TB. tahini (sesame) paste

4 tsp. chia seeds

$^1/_4$ tsp. sea salt

$^1/_4$ tsp. cracked black pepper

2 TB. extra-virgin olive oil

Smoked paprika

1. In a food processor, add chickpeas, lemon juice, garlic, tahini paste, chia seeds, sea salt, black pepper, and 1 tablespoon extra-virgin olive oil and purée until smooth and creamy. Taste and add more lemon juice, garlic, sea salt, or black pepper to your preferred liking.

2. Put in an earthenware bowl, if available, drizzle with remaining 1 tablespoon extra-virgin olive oil, sprinkle with smoked paprika, and serve with sliced vegetables or kale chips.

Chia and Avocado Guacamole

Avocado is the fattiest fruit around, though most people regard it as a vegetable. Luckily, the fats involved are healthy, so you can use the richness of this chia-infused guacamole to help displace fattier foods from your diet while getting lots of good nutrients into your system.

Yield:	Prep time:	Serving size:	
1¹/₂ cups guacamole	10 minutes	about 6 tablespoons guacamole	
Each serving has:			
180 calories	140 calories from fat	16 g total fat	2 g saturated fat
0 mg cholesterol	80 mg sodium	12 g carbohydrates	8 g fiber
1 g sugar	3 g protein	530 mg potassium	40 mg calcium

2 avocados, pit removed and scooped out of skin	2 tsp. chopped garlic
2 scallions, sliced thin	2 TB. chopped cilantro
3 TB. fresh-squeezed lime juice	4 tsp. chia seeds
2 tsp. jalapeño, minced fine	¹/₄ tsp. sea salt
	¹/₄ tsp. cracked black pepper

1. In a medium bowl, place avocados, scallions, lime juice, jalapeño, garlic, cilantro, chia seeds, sea salt, and black pepper and mash until your desired consistency.

2. Serve right away with sliced vegetables or kale chips or refrigerate until ready to serve.

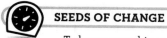 **SEEDS OF CHANGE**

To keep your chia and avocado guacamole from turning brown, place one of the avocado seeds in the prepared mixture until ready to serve.

Cucumber-Chia Raita

Cucumbers are plentiful, inexpensive, filling, and nutritious. This dish adds the smooth, rich flavor of yogurt, the lively spiciness of cilantro, and the tang of lemon to make them more fun to eat.

Yield:	Prep time:	Serving size:	
2 cups raita	20 minutes	$^1/_2$ cup raita	
Each serving has:			
340 calories	220 calories from fat	24 g total fat	18 g saturated fat
40 mg cholesterol	140 mg sodium	13 g carbohydrates	3 g fiber
10 g sugar	17 g protein	28 mg potassium	262 mg calcium

1 qt. whole-milk Greek yogurt

4 tsp. chia seeds

1 tsp. grated lemon zest

$1^1/_2$ tsp. whole cumin seeds, toasted and ground

$^1/_4$ tsp. sea salt

$^1/_4$ tsp. cracked black pepper

2 cucumbers, peeled and deseeded (grate one and dice the other one small)

3 sprigs cilantro

1. In a medium bowl, place whole-milk Greek yogurt, chia seeds, lemon zest, cumin seeds, sea salt and black pepper and mix until smooth.

2. Add cucumbers and cilantro and combine.

3. Chill in the refrigerator until needed and serve with sliced vegetables or kale chips.

Desserts

With all the emphasis in this book on dieting and maintaining a healthy weight, why is there even a chapter on desserts?

For one thing, people love desserts. It's not easy to have a collection of recipes without one—though at least, in this case, they're healthy.

Desserts are also part of a healthy diet. Research has shown that having something sweet at the end of a meal tells your body, "Okay, I'm done." So a small meal and a small dessert may actually be more satisfying than a bigger meal with no dessert.

Westerners, trained to think in a reductionist fashion, simplistically think that "more is more"—that dessert is just more calories, often relatively empty calories, on top of a big meal. But cultures that have been around a long time know how to balance limited resources. So the long-standing tradition of a sweet something—even a glass of sweet wine, such as port—at the end of a meal has wisdom in it.

Chia seeds extend a dessert by helping take up room in your stomach. Drink some water with the chia seeds, and you'll find the treat even more satisfying.

In This Chapter

- Chia pie and cobbler
- Yummy chia cookies
- Chia ices and sorbet
- Chia puddings
- Fun with chia and Jell-O

In addition to the desserts listed in this chapter, you can do a lot of clever things with chia seeds and desserts. Just toss a teaspoon of chia seeds into a cup of sherbet or a dish of Greek yogurt. Or sprinkle chia seeds in a bowl and then add yogurt or sherbet and a few slices of fruit. You're only limited by your imagination, so have fun with it!

 SEEDS OF CHANGE

It's often said that people really only taste the first couple bites of a given dish—after that, the taste buds are more or less on autopilot. So try extra-small servings of dessert, with chia seeds if possible, and a glass of water. Once you've consumed that serving, wait 15 minutes before you decide whether to eat any more.

Chia-Rice Pie

This rice pie has a satisfying, smooth flavor, with sweetness from the honey and a little spiciness from the ricotta cheese.

Yield:	Prep time:	Cook time:	Serving size:
1 pie	20 minutes	45 minutes to 1 hour	1 (about $^1/_2$ cup) slice

Each serving has:			
430 calories	180 calories from fat	20 g total fat	11 g saturated fat
270 mg cholesterol	240 mg sodium	47 g carbohydrates	2 g fiber
32 g sugar	18 g protein	136 mg potassium	257 mg calcium

1 TB. butter

$1^1/_4$ lb. whole-milk ricotta cheese, drained

$^3/_4$ cup raw honey

$^1/_2$ tsp. sea salt

6 eggs

1 tsp. cinnamon

$^1/_2$ tsp. vanilla extract

8 tsp. chia seeds

1 cup cooked rice

1. Preheat the oven to 350°F. Butter a small loaf pan.

2. In a medium bowl, place drained whole-milk ricotta cheese, honey, sea salt, eggs, cinnamon, vanilla extract, and chia seeds and mix until incorporated.

3. Add cooked rice to the bowl, folding in until evenly mixed. Don't overmix.

4. Add mixture to loaf pan and bake for 45 minutes to 1 hour or until golden brown.

5. Cool for 10 minutes before serving.

Blueberry and Chia-Pecan Cobbler

This cobbler gets its richness and chewy texture from the oatmeal and pecans, while the lively flavor of blueberries sends a sweetness.

Yield:	Prep time:	Cook time:	Serving size:
1 cobbler	15 minutes	35 to 40 minutes	1 (1½-cup) slice
Each serving has:			
540 calories	180 calories from fat	21 g total fat	8 g saturated fat
30 mg cholesterol	55 mg sodium	87 g carbohydrates	8 g fiber
54 g sugar	8 g protein	277 mg potassium	53 mg calcium

2 TB. plus ½ stick (¼ cup) butter	¼ tsp. plus pinch sea salt
4 cups fresh blueberries	2 cups oatmeal
1 cup honey	½ cup pecans, chopped
1 TB. lemon zest	2 tsp. ground cinnamon
4 tsp. chia seeds	Pinch sea salt

1. Preheat the oven to 350°F. In a medium saucepan over medium heat, melt 2 tablespoons butter.

2. Stir in blueberries, ¾ cup honey, lemon zest, chia seeds, and ¼ teaspoon sea salt in the saucepan. Turn off flame and incorporate. Pour blueberry mixture into a 4×4-inch pan.

3. In a medium mixing bowl, *cream* together remaining ½ stick butter, remaining ¼ cup honey, and oatmeal. Once ingredients are incorporated, add pecans, cinnamon, and remaining pinch sea salt. Crumble pecan mixture evenly over blueberry mixture.

4. Bake cobbler for 35 to 40 minutes, until topping is golden brown and a fork stuck into the topping comes out clean.

5. Let cobbler cool to room temperature before serving.

 DEFINITION

To **cream** ingredients together means to mix them until they're smooth. It's an expression that's most often used with creamy ingredients, such as butter or cream cheese. The idea is that you keep mixing until the ingredients being added to the creamy ingredient are thoroughly blended in.

Chia Pizzelles

Pizzelles add the mild sweetness of sugar to the rich and savory flavor of baked eggs.

Yield:	Prep time:	Cook time:	Serving size:
18 pizzelles	20 minutes	30 minutes	3 pizzelles

Each serving has:			
360 calories	160 calories from fat	18 g total fat	10 g saturated fat
150 mg cholesterol	35 mg sodium	37 g carbohydrates	11 g fiber
22 g sugar	10 g protein	5 mg potassium	228 mg calcium

$^1/_4$ lb. unsalted butter	$1^1/_3$ cups chia flour
3 eggs	$^2/_3$ cup granulated sugar
$^1/_2$ tsp. vanilla extract	

1. In a small saucepan over medium-high heat, melt butter, being careful not to brown it. Let cool to room temperature but not until solidified.

2. Mix in eggs, vanilla extract, chia flour, and sugar with a whisk.

3. Preheat a pizzelle iron to high. Ladle in a sample of batter, about ¾ cup, until you find the right amount for your particular pizzelle iron. Cook pizzelles until brown.

4. Serve warm. If you're saving them for later, allow pizzelles to cool in a single layer; don't stack them until completely cool.

 SEEDS OF CHANGE

If you don't have a pizzelle iron, you can use a frying pan and treat them like you're making pancakes. However, you should cover the pizzelle with a saucepan top during cooking to get a baking effect.

Flourless Chia-Peanut Butter Cookies

Yield:	Prep time:	Cook time:	Serving size:
12 cookies	12 minutes	10 minutes	2 cookies

Each serving has:			
410 calories	210 calories from fat	23 g total fat	4 g saturated fat
35 mg cholesterol	430 mg sodium	45 g carbohydrates	5 g fiber
36 g sugar	12 g protein	343 mg potassium	44 mg calcium

1 cup chunky peanut butter

$^3/_4$ cup honey

1 egg, beaten

1 tsp. baking soda

$^1/_4$ tsp. vanilla extract

6 tsp. chia seeds

1. Preheat the oven to 350°F. Grease a baking sheet.

2. In a medium bowl, beat together peanut butter and honey with an electric hand mixer until smooth and creamy. Add beaten egg, baking soda, vanilla extract, and chia seeds and mix until ingredients are combined.

3. Quickly roll out teaspoon-sized balls of dough and place an inch apart from one another on the baking sheet. Flatten dough balls with a fork.

4. Bake cookies until golden color and puffy, about 10 minutes.

5. Cool and serve topped with your favorite fruit jam for a classic peanut-butter-and-jelly taste.

Chia-Blackberry Ice

Ices are smooth and often delicious. This one, which gets its flavor from blackberries, is sweet and tangy. You can try the same recipe with other kinds of berries as well.

Yield:	Prep time:	Freeze time:	Serving size:
1 pt. ice	10 minutes	about 6 hours	3 oz. ice

Each serving has:			
70 calories	10 calories from fat	1 g total fat	0 g saturated fat
0 mg cholesterol	0 mg sodium	17 g carbohydrates	3 g fiber
13 g sugar	1 g protein	16 mg potassium	28 mg calcium

1 pt. fresh, ripe blackberries or other berries	2 TB. lemon juice
1/2 cup water	1/2 tsp. lemon zest
4 TB. honey	4 tsp. chia seeds

1. In a blender, place blackberries, water, honey, lemon juice, lemon zest, and chia seeds and blend on low speed until completely mixed.

2. Pour mixture into a shallow pan with a lid and freeze, mixing thoroughly every half hour for first couple of hours. Replace lid and freeze overnight.

3. If the ice is too solid to serve, remove from the freezer and let sit at room temperature for about 10 or 15 minutes until easily scraped with a scoop.

Blackberry-Merlot-Chia Ice

This simple dish adds the smooth, sophisticated flavor of merlot to the sweet richness of blackberries, along with the nutritional kick of chia seeds.

Yield:	Prep time:	Cook time:	Serving size:
2 cups ice	4 hours	10 minutes	$^1/_2$ cup ice

Each serving has:			
160 calories	15 calories from fat	1.5 g total fat	0 g saturated fat
0 mg cholesterol	0 mg sodium	34 g carbohydrates	8 g fiber
25 g sugar	3 g protein	280 mg potassium	64 mg calcium

4 cups blackberries	4 tsp. chia seeds
$^3/_4$ cup water	1 TB. lemon juice
$^1/_2$ cup sugar	1 cinnamon stick
$^1/_2$ cup merlot	

1. In a large bowl, combine blackberries, water, sugar, merlot, chia seeds, lemon juice, and cinnamon stick.

2. In a medium saucepan over medium-high heat, bring mixture to a boil, stirring occasionally.

3. Remove from heat and let stand for 15 minutes.

4. Pour into a glass bowl, place in the freezer, and freeze for 4 hours, stirring every hour.

5. Remove from the freezer, spoon into bowls, and serve.

Dark Chocolate–Chia Pudding

Dark chocolate has a rich, smoky flavor that's intriguing, so much so that you don't need to add a lot of sweetener to make a dark chocolate dish attractive. Using almond milk keeps the calorie count of this dish down.

Yield:	Prep time:	Serving size:	
3 cups pudding	5 to 8 hours	$^3/_4$ cup pudding	
Each serving has:			
150 calories	80 calories from fat	9 g total fat	1 g saturated fat
0 mg cholesterol	140 mg sodium	16 g carbohydrates	9 g fiber
5 g sugar	5 g protein	175 mg potassium	272 mg calcium

3 cups unsweetened almond milk	2 pkt. stevia
$^1/_2$ cup chia seeds	1 TB. honey
3 TB. dark cocoa powder	

1. In a medium bowl, whisk together unsweetened almond milk, chia seeds, dark cocoa powder, stevia, and honey.

2. Cover and refrigerate for 5 hours or overnight.

3. Serve.

 SEEDS OF CHANGE

You can use other milks instead of unsweetened almond milk, such as skim dairy milk, soy milk, and rice milk. You can also garnish the pudding with shaved chocolate, whipped cream, or whipped soy.

Chocolate-Chia Pudding

The sweet, rich taste of chocolate pudding makes for a fun way to enjoy the goodness of chia. This version uses almond milk instead of dairy milk to reduce calories and fat, with the added chia seeds providing the thickness.

Yield:	Prep time:	Cook time:	Serving size:
2 cups pudding	5 minutes	10 minutes	$^1/_2$ cup pudding

Each serving has:			
210 calories	100 calories from fat	11 g total fat	6 g saturated fat
5 mg cholesterol	60 mg sodium	31 g carbohydrates	4 g fiber
16 g sugar	1 g protein	75 mg potassium	40 mg calcium

1$^1/_2$ cups almond milk	$^1/_2$ cup dark chocolate chips
4 tsp. cornstarch	1 tsp. unsalted butter
2 TB. granulated sugar	$^1/_2$ tsp. vanilla extract
2 TB. chia seeds	

1. In a bowl, whisk together almond milk, cornstarch, sugar, and chia seeds.

2. Pour mixture into a medium saucepan and bring just to a boil over medium-high heat.

3. Lower heat to medium and whisk 3 to 4 minutes until thickened.

4. Turn off heat. Add dark chocolate chips, butter, and vanilla extract and whisk until smooth.

5. Serve warm, or cover with plastic wrap and chill before serving.

 SEEDS OF CHANGE

Note that each teaspoonful of this pudding only has about 7 calories and less than 1 gram of fat. Adding it to fruit is a delicious way to create a balanced dessert.

Banana-Chia Pudding

Sometimes you want to go all out and have a rich dessert. This dessert combines the smooth, rich flavors of bananas and cream with the crunch of vanilla wafers.

Yield:	Prep time:	Cook time:	Serving size:
4 bowls pudding	5 minutes	10 minutes	1 bowl pudding

Each serving has:			
360 calories	130 calories from fat	14 g total fat	6 g saturated fat
110 mg cholesterol	180 mg sodium	58 g carbohydrates	7 g fiber
33 g sugar	7 g protein	504 mg potassium	121 mg calcium

³/₄ cup half and half	Pinch sea salt
1 large egg yolk	¹/₂ TB. unsalted butter
¹/₄ cup sugar	1 tsp. vanilla extract
2 tsp. cornstarch	4 medium bananas
2 TB. chia seeds	12 vanilla wafers, broken

1. In a medium bowl, whisk together half and half, egg yolk, sugar, cornstarch, chia seeds, and sea salt.

2. Pour into a medium saucepan and bring to a boil over medium-high heat.

3. Turn off heat and whisk in butter and vanilla extract.

4. Slice 2 bananas and place in the bottom of serving cups or bowls. Sprinkle in half of broken vanilla wafers among each.

5. Pour half of pudding over bananas and wafers.

6. Slice remaining 2 bananas and place over first half of pudding. Sprinkle remaining broken vanilla wafers among each.

7. Pour remaining half of pudding over bananas and wafers and serve.

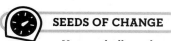 **SEEDS OF CHANGE**

You can bulk up the nutrition of this dessert with additional fresh fruit.

Chia-Jell-O and Applesauce Salad

Applesauce has a rich and spicy taste, while Jell-O has a bouncy texture that serves as a good medium for chia seeds.

Yield:	Prep time:	Cook time:	Serving size:
3 cups salad	2 hours	10 minutes	$^1/_2$ cup salad

Each serving has:			
60 calories	10 calories from fat	1 g total fat	0 g saturated fat
0 mg cholesterol	0 mg sodium	11 g carbohydrates	2 g fiber
8 g sugar	2 g protein	65 mg potassium	23 mg calcium

1 cup water	2 TB. chia seeds
1 pkg. strawberry Jell-O	2 cups applesauce

1. In a medium saucepan over high heat, bring water to a boil.

2. Stir in strawberry Jell-O and chia seeds and remove the saucepan from the heat.

3. Pour mixture into a medium bowl and add applesauce.

4. Chill until set, about 2 hours. Serve.

Vegan Gelatin with Chia

You may not know it, but most gelatin—including commercial Jell-O—is made from animals. This version uses kanten powder, also known as agar agar. It's a combination of sea plants, available in health food stores and elsewhere. Like chia, it leaves you feeling full, even if you don't eat much.

Yield:	Prep time:	Cook time:	Serving size:
4 cups gelatin	2 hours	10 minutes	1 cup gelatin
Each serving has:			
25 calories	15 calories from fat	1.5 g total fat	0 g saturated fat
0 mg cholesterol	0 mg sodium	3 g carbohydrates	2 g fiber
0 g sugar	1 g protein	13 mg potassium	30 mg calcium

4 cups water	2 TB. chia seeds
2 TB. kanten powder	2 tsp. stevia

1. In a medium bowl, combine water, kanten powder, and chia seeds.

2. Pour into a medium saucepan, cover, and bring to a boil over medium-high heat.

3. Reduce heat to medium and simmer for 5 minutes.

4. Add stevia and pour into a glass bowl or baking dish.

5. Place in the refrigerator and chill for at least 2 hours, stirring after 30 minutes to stop chia seeds from settling to the bottom.

6. Remove from the refrigerator and serve.

 SEEDS OF CHANGE

> As with all of these desserts, you can garnish this vegan gelatin dish with Greek yogurt to add visual variety, sweetness, and a creamy texture.

Low-Fat Chocolate Sorbet with Chia

Chocolate is so sweet, it's hard to believe that a rich sorbet can be so low in calories—and so rich in chia goodness!

Yield:	Prep time:	Cook time:	Serving size:
4 cups sorbet	2 hours	10 minutes	$^1/_2$ cup sorbet

Each serving has:			
150 calories	60 calories from fat	7 g total fat	4.5 g saturated fat
0 mg cholesterol	0 mg sodium	29 g carbohydrates	4 g fiber
23 g sugar	2 g protein	85 mg potassium	21 mg calcium

$2^1/_2$ cups water	2 TB. chia seeds
1 cup granulated sugar	4 oz. bittersweet chocolate
$^1/_2$ cup unsweetened cocoa powder	2 tsp. vanilla extract

1. In a medium saucepan over high heat, bring water to a boil.

2. Stir in sugar, unsweetened cocoa powder, and chia seeds.

3. Reduce heat to medium and simmer for 5 minutes, stirring occasionally.

4. Add bittersweet chocolate and vanilla extract and stir for 2 minutes. Turn off heat.

5. Pour into a large bowl, cover, and freeze for about 2 hours.

6. Scoop into bowls and serve.

Glossary

al dente   Italian for "against the teeth," this term refers to pasta or rice that's neither soft nor hard but just slightly firm against the teeth.

bake   To cook in a dry oven. Dry-heat cooking often results in a crisping of the exterior of the food being cooked. Moist-heat cooking—through methods such as steaming, poaching, and so on—brings a much different, moist quality to the food.

baking powder   A dry ingredient used to increase volume and lighten or leaven baked goods.

balsamic vinegar   Vinegar produced primarily in Italy from a specific type of grape and aged in wood barrels. It's heavier, darker, and sweeter than most vinegars.

basil   A flavorful, almost sweet, resinous herb delicious with tomatoes and used in all kinds of Italian- and Mediterranean-style dishes.

beat   To quickly mix substances.

blacken   To cook something quickly in a very hot skillet over high heat, usually with a seasoning mixture.

blend   To completely mix something, usually with a blender or food processor, slower than beating.

boil   To heat a liquid to the point where water is forced to turn into steam, causing the liquid to bubble. To boil something is to insert it into boiling water. A rapid boil is when a lot of bubbles form on the surface of the liquid.

brown   To cook in a skillet, turning, until the food's surface is seared and brown in color, to lock in the juices.

brown rice   A whole-grain rice, including the germ, with a characteristic pale brown or tan color. It's more nutritious and flavorful than white rice.

bruschetta (or **crostini**)   Slices of toasted or grilled bread with garlic and olive oil, often with other toppings.

caper   The flavorful buds of a Mediterranean plant, ranging in size from *nonpareil* (about the size of a small pea) to larger, grape-size caper berries produced in Spain.

caramelize   To cook sugar over low heat until it develops a sweet caramel flavor, or to cook vegetables (especially onions) or meat in butter or oil over low heat until they soften, sweeten, and develop a caramel color.

chia seed   The tiny white or black seed of the chia plant, which comes from the sage family.

chickpea (or **garbanzo bean**)   A roundish yellow-gold bean used as the base ingredient in hummus. Chickpeas are high in fiber and low in fat.

chile (or **chili**)   Any one of many different "hot" peppers, ranging in intensity from the relatively mild ancho pepper to the blisteringly hot habanero.

chili powder   A warm, rich seasoning blend that includes chile pepper, cumin, garlic, and oregano.

chop   To cut into pieces, usually qualified by an adverb such as "*coarsely* chopped" or by a size measurement such as "chopped into ½-inch pieces." "Finely chopped" is much closer to mince.

cilantro   A member of the parsley family used in Mexican dishes (especially salsa) and some Asian dishes. Use in moderation, because the flavor can overwhelm. The seed of the cilantro plant is the spice coriander.

curry   Rich, spicy, Indian-style sauces and the dishes prepared with them. A curry uses curry powder as its base seasoning.

deglaze   To scrape up bits of meat and seasoning left in a pan or skillet after cooking. Usually this is done by adding a liquid such as wine or broth and creating a flavorful stock that can be used to create sauces.

Dijon mustard   A hearty, spicy mustard made in the style of the Dijon region of France.

double boiler   A set of two pots designed to nest together, one inside the other, and provide consistent, moist heat for foods that need delicate treatment. The bottom pot holds water (not quite touching the bottom of the top pot); the top pot holds the food you want to heat.

frittata   A skillet-cooked mixture of eggs and other ingredients that's not stirred but is cooked slowly and then either flipped or finished under the broiler.

fry   *See* sauté.

garlic   A member of the onion family, a pungent and flavorful vegetable used in many savory dishes. A garlic bulb contains multiple cloves. Each clove, when chopped, provides about 1 teaspoon garlic.

ginger   A flavorful root available fresh or dried and ground that adds a pungent, sweet, and spicy quality to a dish.

Greek yogurt   A strained yogurt that's a good natural source of protein, calcium, and probiotics. Greek yogurt averages 40 percent more protein per ounce than traditional yogurt.

hummus   A thick, Middle Eastern spread made of puréed chickpeas, lemon juice, olive oil, garlic, and often tahini.

julienne   A French word meaning "to slice into very thin pieces."

kombucha   Originally found in Central Asia, but now popular worldwide, it is a drink made by fermenting tea. Usually served at room temperature or chilled, not hot.

meld   To allow flavors to blend and spread over time. Melding is often why recipes call for overnight refrigeration and is also why some dishes taste better as leftovers.

mouthfeel   The overall sensation in the mouth resulting from a combination of a food's temperature, taste, smell, and texture.

nutmeg   A sweet, fragrant, musky spice used primarily in baking.

olive   The fruit of the olive tree commonly grown on all sides of the Mediterranean. Black olives are also called ripe olives. Green olives are immature, although they're also widely eaten.

olive oil   A fragrant liquid produced by crushing or pressing olives. Extra-virgin olive oil—the most flavorful and highest quality—is produced from the first pressing of a batch of olives; oil is also produced from later pressings.

oregano   A fragrant, slightly astringent herb used in Greek, Spanish, and Italian dishes.

oxidation   The browning of fruit flesh that happens over time and with exposure to air. Minimize oxidation by rubbing the cut surfaces with lemon juice.

pesto   A thick spread or sauce made with fresh basil leaves, garlic, olive oil, pine nuts, and Parmesan cheese.

pilaf   A rice dish in which the rice is browned in butter or oil and then cooked in a flavorful liquid such as a broth, often with the addition of meats or vegetables. The rice absorbs the broth, resulting in a savory dish.

pinch   An unscientific measurement for the amount of an ingredient—typically, a dry, granular substance such as an herb or seasoning—you can hold between your finger and thumb.

pine nut   A nut that's rich (high in fat), flavorful, and a bit pine-y. Pine nuts are a traditional ingredient in pesto and add a hearty crunch to many other recipes.

quinoa   A nutty-flavored seed that's extremely high in protein and calcium.

reduce   To boil or simmer a broth or sauce to remove some of the water content, resulting in more concentrated flavor and color.

render   To cook a meat to the point where its fat melts and can be removed.

reserve   To hold a specified ingredient for another use later in the recipe.

roast   To cook something uncovered in an oven, usually without additional liquid.

sauté   To pan-cook over lower heat than what's used for frying.

savory   A popular herb with a fresh, woody taste. Can also describe the flavor of food.

sear   To quickly brown the exterior of a food, especially meat, over high heat.

shellfish   A broad range of seafood, including clams, mussels, oysters, crabs, shrimp, and lobster.

simmer   To boil a liquid gently so it barely bubbles.

skillet (also **frying pan**)   A generally heavy, flat-bottomed, metal pan with a handle designed to cook food over heat on a stovetop or campfire.

steam   To suspend a food over boiling water and allow the heat of the steam (water vapor) to cook the food. This quick-cooking method preserves a food's flavor and texture.

stir-fry   To cook small pieces of food in a wok or skillet over high heat, moving and turning the food quickly to cook all sides.

tempeh   An Indonesian food made by culturing and fermenting soybeans into a cake, sometimes mixed with grains or vegetables. It's high in protein and fiber.

thyme   A minty, zesty herb.

vinegar   An acidic liquid widely used as a dressing and seasoning, often made from fermented grapes, apples, or rice. *See also* balsamic vinegar; white vinegar; wine vinegar.

whisk   To rapidly mix, introducing air to the mixture.

white mushroom   A button mushroom. When fresh, white mushrooms have an earthy smell and an appealing soft crunch.

white vinegar   The most common type of vinegar, produced from grain.

whole grain   A grain derived from the seeds of grasses, including rice, oats, rye, wheat, wild rice, quinoa, barley, buckwheat, bulgur, corn, millet, amaranth, and sorghum.

whole-wheat flour   Wheat flour that contains the entire grain.

wine vinegar   Vinegar produced from red or white wine.

zest   Small slivers of peel, usually from a citrus fruit such as a lemon, lime, or orange.

Resources

There are a lot of resources available about chia. Luckily, chia is a rare enough word that most of the "hits" you get online have at least some relationship to improving your diet using chia seeds. But you'll also find oddities—such as the Chia Pet, of course, and one Mantuk Chia, author of many books about spirituality and intimate relations. In this appendix, we give you paper and online resources to help you get straight to information about chia seeds and your diet.

Because you've already put down good money for this book, we made sure all the online sources we mention are free to use. (Though some of them, such as online shops with chia products, give you additional ways to spend money!)

Books

There are quite a few books about chia out there. Here are three of the most popular ones:

Arnot, Bob. *The Aztec Diet: Chia Power: The Superfood That Gets You Skinny and Keeps You Healthy.* New York: William Morrow, 2013.

Bob Arnot is a doctor and a big chia booster, and this book shows his enthusiasm. He attributes much of the success of the Aztec empire to chia—which, unfortunately, is something we can't actually know—and recommends that you start out by including three chia shakes a day in your diet. This book will teach you a lot about chia, but this is one case where it can't hurt to take your chia (or this chia book, anyway) with a grain of salt.

Coates, Wayne. *Chia: The Complete Guide to the Ultimate Superfood.* New York: Sterling, 2012.

Dr. Coates is an early and effective proponent of chia seeds. Like Dr. Arnot, he ties chia strongly to the Aztecs. While this book is a bit on the short side, it's full of recipes and good advice on using chia.

MySeeds Chia Test Kitchen. *The Chia Seed Cookbook: Eat Well, Feel Great, Lose Weight.* New York: Skyhorse Publishing, 2013.

This book provides lots of recipes and beautiful photographs. It's somewhat lacking in theory, which can make it harder to use chia in your already-favorite recipes and to keep including chia in your diet over the long haul. But if you're looking to expand your chia recipe collection, this is a nice resource.

Presentations

If you know people who find the idea of reading a whole book about chia seeds a bit intimidating, or if you just need some short and to-the-point information about chia, there are several presentations online about the goodness of chia, such as the following. You can also share this information with friends or colleagues as a source of inspiration.

Chia: The Super Food of the Ancient Aztecs

issacharenterprises.net/index%20files/Chia.htm

Issachar Enterprises, which offers a branded chia seed product called Omega3 Chia, has a presentation that sums up many of the best points about chia seeds. On this page, you can also find a link to the presentation in PowerPoint format.

PDF Documents

There are many PDFs available about chia seeds. Much of the material is already covered in this book, but there's more official, scientific, and in-depth information in some of them you may find useful.

Some of the PDFs also have chia-infused recipes. There are more than 100 recipes in this book, but when it comes to recipes, too much is never enough!

Chia Plant Guide from the USDA

plants.usda.gov/plantguide/pdf/cs_sac06.pdf

This PDF from the U.S. Department of Agriculture's Natural Resources Conservation Service includes a scientific description of the plant, its habitat, and how to grow chia yourself. It also features some good references.

Chia Seed Nutrition and Uses from OriginalFastFoods.com

api.ning.com/files/jczvfQFfii6n3LGqvRZfyydiq*QPtZTTXXi9rOetqQ5okXJCaKx9y4ptX-i80J4z7vHF2d2zRXeBM3lwv195JAEl4wAGLQM4/chiadressingsdips.pdf

This is a well-written summary of chia seed information with a small number of recipes, including a few particularly useful "core" recipes. The site is organized around the useful idea that you can get the convenience of fast food from "real," healthy foods—a viewpoint we heartily endorse.

Chia Seeds: The Aztec Wonder Food from the Center for Integrative Health

www.cih.nusystem.org/assets/resources/pageResources/ithrive-023.pdf

This is a beautifully formatted six-page brochure on the benefits of chia. It's not all that deep, but if you need a glossy presentation to show someone who values style as much as substance (or even a bit more), go no further. This also includes two recipes you can try.

Chia Seeds from GoodCause Wellness

goodcausewellness.com/chia_seed_recipes_gcw.pdf

This PDF gives some introduction to how chia seeds work, along with really detailed nutritional information. You can also find a number of useful recipes in this document.

Chia Seeds Ebook from Natural Healthy Choices

naturalhealthychoices.ca/resources/NHC%20Ebook-Chia%20Seeds%20Health%20Benefits%20and%20Recipes.pdf

This chia seeds ebook is a well-formatted, 16-page summary of chia and its benefits. The site that the report was developed for has a praiseworthy mission statement: "We specialize in gluten free low, glycemic organic foods and high performance nutraceuticals that aid and promote daily nutritional support, wellness and healthier life style."

Market and Growing Information from the University of Kentucky

uky.edu/Ag/CDBREC/introsheets/chia.pdf

Like many colleges with agriculture departments, the University of Kentucky runs an extension service to provide farmers with information. This concise, well-formatted, three-page report gives an introduction to chia for farmers considering planting it. The report is not for farmers only, though—the perspective is fascinating, and the resource links at the end are worth following up on.

Technical Details from the National Science Research Institute

nsrinews.com/abstracts/Chia_Technical_Sheet.pdf

The National Science Research Institute (NSRI), a nonprofit that provides nutritional information and certification, has a PDF with detailed technical information about chia. My favorite part is a page comparing chia to fish oil, algae, and flax. (Hint: Chia comes out on top.) The report also says that chia seeds are kosher!

Index

C

E

F

S

T

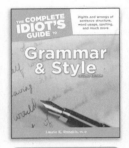
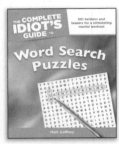
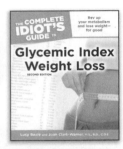
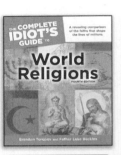
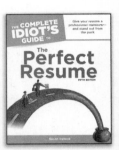
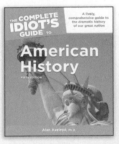
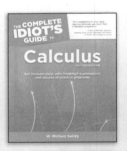
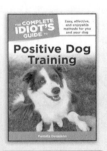
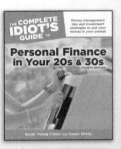
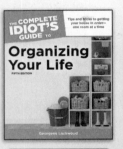
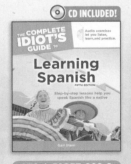
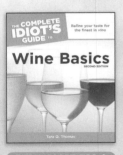
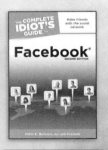
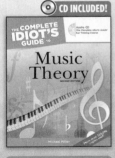
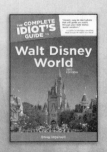